ANTI-INFLAMMATORY DIET IN THE ERA OF COVID-19

Dean M. Toriumi, MD.

Copyright © 2020 by DMT Solutions

All rights reserved.
No part of this publication may be reproduced, stored in a retrieval system, or transmitted in any form or by any means, mechanical, photocopying, recording, or otherwise without prior permission of the publisher.
The owner, publisher, and editor are not responsible
for errors and omissions.

Limit of Liability/Disclosure of Warranty: Please note that this advice is generic and not specific to any individual. You should consult with your doctor before undertaking any medical or nutritional course of action.

Publisher: DMT Solutions
Production Services: DMT Solutions
Editorial: Patricia Stahl
Illustrator: Bridget Gillespie and Karen Mitchell
Layout: Open Look Business Solutions, Inc.

Dean M. Toriumi, MD
Anti-inflammatory Diet in the Era of Covid-19/Dean M. Toriumi, MD
Chicago: DMT Solutions, 2020

Includes bibliographical references and index.

ISBN 978-1-7357004-0-3

Printed in the United States

Table of Contents

iv	**DEDICATION**
v	**FOREWORD**
ix	**PREFACE**
xiv	**ACKNOWLEDGMENTS**
xv	**INTRODUCTION**
1	**CHAPTER 1:** Your Nose, Sinuses and Immune System —The First Line of Defense Against COVID-19
11	**CHAPTER 2:** The Glycemic Index and Inflammation
17	**CHAPTER 3:** Anti-inflammatory Foods—The Key to Managing Your Body's Inflammation
44	**CHAPTER 4:** Olive Oil and Its Importance in the Anti-inflammatory Diet
53	**CHAPTER 5:** Green Tea and Supplements
67	**CHAPTER 6:** The Impact of Exercise on Your Immune System and Covid-19 Outcome
76	**CHAPTER 7:** Your Waistline Tells the Story
84	**CHAPTER 8:** Anti-inflammatory Diet with Keto Push
98	**CHAPTER 9:** Effects of Anti-inflammatory Diet on Your Skin and Aging
105	**CHAPTER 10:** Arthritis, Back Pain and the Anti-inflammatory Diet
110	**CHAPTER 11:** Practical Ways to Incorporate the Anti-inflammatory Diet
127	**CHAPTER 12:** Different Anti-inflammatory Diet Plans Based on Your Goals
163	**CHAPTER 13:** Inflammation and Covid-19
173	**CHAPTER 14:** Clinical Experience with the Anti-inflammatory Diet
182	**CHAPTER 15:** Patient Experiences with the Anti-inflammatory Diet
189	**CHAPTER 16:** Final Thoughts: Learning to Live with Coronavirus

Dedication

I dedicate this book to my wife and friend, Colleen, who helped me write the book and determine what information would be most useful to the reader. She has supported my efforts in developing this diet plan for decreasing inflammation.

I also dedicate this book to Hannah, Jesse, Olivia and Joe; to my parents, John and Kay; and to those health care workers who were on the front lines during the Covid-19 pandemic.

Foreword

The book entitled *Anti-inflammatory Diet in the Era of Covid-19* is a must read for those of you who would like to take charge and improve your chances of beating Covid-19 should it come back again. We can do this by preventing, improving or eliminating illnesses such as hypertension, heart disease, diabetes, asthma and obesity, which could make you more vulnerable to the coronavirus.

And the benefits range far beyond that! Maybe you want to improve your allergies, minimize your back pain or simply create a healthier overall version of yourself. This is all possible by decreasing your body's inflammation. Yes, you are likely inflamed, and that is contributing to your runny nose, your painful joints, your red skin tone or your general lethargy. This is a great time to learn about the anti-inflammatory diet and how you can make modifications in your diet, decrease your body's inflammation and bolster your immune system.

Dean and I have known each other for many years. Both of us are rhinoplasty surgeons who make a living fixing people's noses. This is a very complex operation and requires a great deal of attention to detail, precision in execution and long surgeries. In order to accomplish this, both Dean and I exercise almost every day and try to keep fit. We need a strong core to allow us to perform these long operations. We both eat well (that's the hardest part for me) in order to stay fit and maximize our ability to perform in surgery. This all starts with a healthy diet. I have known Dean for years, and everyone talks about his diet. We'll be at meetings together and he always eats differently than the rest of us. Many of us have always wanted to know the details behind his quirky diet.

In this book, Dean clearly describes the anti-inflammatory diet and how you can incorporate it into your daily lifestyle. This diet is not a fad and is something that you can incorporate into your daily routine. In his book, Dean starts out explaining why the anti-inflammatory diet is important to those of you who would like to improve your general health. More importantly, beyond Covid-19, Dean will tell you how you can improve your general health to feel better, perform better and potentially live longer.

After introducing the anti-inflammatory diet at the beginning of the book, he goes into the philosophy and science behind the diet. He goes into specifics about dietary choices including meal options for breakfast, lunch and dinner. He explains what are inflammatory foods, neutral foods and anti-inflammatory foods. You will be surprised at what those simple carbs are doing to your blood sugar and your immune system. Dean additionally explains how the Covid-19 virus likely comes into your body through your nose. He discusses your nasal anatomy and how your nose can be prepared to better fight off the virus if some particles enter your nasal cavity. He also discusses important supplements that can strengthen your immune system and help you prevent viral infection. He clearly explains how you can strengthen your immune system by controlling your diet. Eating anti-inflammatory foods such as spinach, broccoli and avocado; taking supplements (green tea, curcumin, olive oil, etc.); and exercising will strengthen your immune system. This is the core of the book and the immune system boost is what may help protect you from the coronavirus. The discussion on green tea in itself is quite extensive and will likely entice you to drink a couple of cups a day.

I really enjoyed reading the chapters on exercise, your waistline and the keto push. These topics are right up my alley. In this chapter of my life, staying fit and looking great are important to me. This is particularly important with our television show,

"Botched," performing well. I also have a new beautiful wife and a baby girl on the way. I need to be young at heart and have the heart of a young man as well.

I really like how Dean explains everything clearly in layman's terms with the most important points being referenced. The concept of an anti-inflammatory diet with the keto push is really innovative and will be interesting to even younger readers who may not be that concerned with Covid-19. The keto component is key to decreasing your body fat and trimming your mid-section. A big waist is a bad indicator for heart disease, diabetes and an early departure from this world. When you look at this book, it is evident it was written in the time of Covid-19 as it has a coronavirus focus; however, the content is great for anyone who is just interested in living a healthy lifestyle and would like to look and feel great. You could change the title and remove the references to Covid-19 and this book would still be just as beneficial. Personally, I read it without the same concern about the coronavirus as many my age but got a lot out of it despite my different focus.

You may ask, why read a book on the anti-inflammatory diet by a rhinoplasty surgeon? Well, I can tell you Dean obviously has done a lot of research on this topic. I would consider Dean an expert on the anti-inflammatory diet. He has been into this diet for over 20 years. He's studied it and has practiced it on a daily basis for that same period of time. He also garnered a tremendous amount of data by promoting the diet to his patients. This is the key behind his level of expertise on the topic. Being a physician and surgeon, he has treated many patients who were inflamed and became less inflamed on the diet. He has recommended the anti-inflammatory diet to many of his patients over the years and has accumulated extensive clinical experience with the prescribing of the diet. He also completed a clinical study on the anti-inflammatory diet, demonstrating improvement in the patient's symptoms (nasal symptoms, back pain, joint pain, etc.).

Dean's experience with the anti-inflammatory diet is clear when you read the book.

I am excited that Dean has written this book to help others who would like to live a healthy lifestyle and potentially extend their lifespan. He has chosen an opportune time to release the book when many are looking to improve their health in this Covid-19 era.

I highly recommend that you take a look at Dean's book and read it with the coronavirus in mind, but also if you would like to improve yourself. Only you can make the change, and now is the time!

Paul S. Nassif, MD.
Facial Plastic Surgery
"Star of E!'s Botched"

Preface

The "novel coronavirus" is also known as severe acute respiratory syndrome coronavirus 2 or SARS-CoV-2. Once infected by SARS-CoV-2, some may develop a deadly respiratory disease called Covid-19.

SARS-CoV-2 hit the United States in early 2020, infecting many Americans and killing more than 150,000 *(App P-1 Ref. To access this and subsequent references, go to Google Play Store or Apple App Store and purchase a subscription for the app for this book.)* Most of those who died from Covid-19 were older than 65 years of age *(App P-2 Ref.)*.[1] Of those who died, 76.4% had at least one underlying medical condition (comorbidity). The most common underlying medical conditions were obesity *(App P-3 Ref.)*, heart disease and diabetes.

Many experts believed the Covid-19 pandemic would decline during the summer months. In reality, the virus rebounded during the summer in many states with increased numbers of hospitalizations and deaths. There are fears that the virus will reemerge with vigor in the fall and winter of 2020, extending into 2021. Other than social distancing, wearing face coverings and washing our hands, many think we are limited in what we can do to protect ourselves against the coronvirus.

Many entities are working on a vaccine to treat Covid-19 and one may be available in late 2020 or early 2021. Most first generation vaccines will not make you immune to the virus but may make you less likely to have a bad outcome. Additionally, many are concerned about the safety of these new vaccines. Bottom line, the early vaccines will likely not completely protect you from getting infected.

The SARS-CoV-2 enters the body primarily through the nose and ultimately attacks the lungs. Once the virus reaches the lungs, the body launches an inflammatory response against the virus that may actually cause severe damage. The lungs tend to fill with inflammatory cells and fluid, making breathing difficult. This may lead to the need for a ventilator. This response is due to increased inflammation and a damaging "self-directed" response by the person's immune system. By decreasing inflammation, this inflammatory response can be dampened. The mechanism of progression of the disease through inflammation in the lungs is supported by the effective use of corticosteroids to treat patients that are having severe lung problems *(App P-4 Ref.)*. Corticosteroids help to decrease inflammation in the lungs and decrease the damaging response to the lungs.

The strength of your immune system may be one of the most important defenses that your body has to prevent infection by SARS-CoV-2. When the virus enters your body, it must attach to receptors in your nasal lining, throat, lungs, eyes, etc., to enter your body.[2] If your immune system is strong, infection-fighting cells in your body may be able to fight off the virus and prevent infection. This means that some individuals with a strong immune system may be exposed to the SARS-CoV-2 virus but are able to fight off the exposure and not get infected, whereas others with a weaker immune system may be exposed to the same virus and need to be hospitalized.

I wrote this book in part to give you a means to strengthen your own internal defenses to protect yourself against this potentially recurring virus. The strategy is to decrease the inflammation, strengthen your immune system and decrease or eliminate your underlying medical disorders. However, the purpose of the book goes far beyond the impact of Covid-19. I have been a strong supporter of this diet for many years and wanted to provide as much information as possible for everyone interested in getting healthier.

The anti-inflammatory diet has been around for many years and is based on the premise that everything you eat and drink is either inflammatory, anti-inflammatory or neutral (neither pro-inflammatory nor anti-inflammatory). In this book I will give you the information that you will need to pick foods that will decrease your body's inflammation. By decreasing your body's inflammation, you will decrease the likelihood of a bad outcome if you should contract Covid-19 *(App P-5 Ref.)*. I will also discuss supplements that you can take to help strengthen your immune system. The goal is to make your immune system strong again so you can fight off the virus like those younger people who tend to be asymptomatic when they contract the virus. I also go into detail about other lifestyle changes that you can institute to further strengthen your immune system. These include exercising, improving your mood, getting better sleep and decreasing stress in your life.

The other goal of instituting the anti-inflammatory diet will be to avoid or lessen the severity of your medical conditions. It is clear that people who have medical problems such as obesity, heart disease, diabetes, kidney disease and lung diseases such as asthma have a much higher risk to experience a poor outcome or death if they should contract Covid-19.[3] You can help to prevent or lessen the severity of these medical conditions if you go on an anti-inflammatory diet.[4][5]

Obesity is one of the most significant medical problems that sets you up for a poor outcome if you contract Covid-19 *(App P-6 Ref.)*. Increased girth in your midsection may indicate that you have an excessive amount of visceral fat (fat in your abdominal cavity) that can cause inflammation *(App P-7 Ref.)*.[6] The visceral fat may also be associated with weakening of your immune system *(App P-8 Ref.)*. One of the most popular means to decrease your body's fat is to incorporate the keto diet. The keto diet has been shown to quickly shed visceral fat and decrease the girth of your midsection *(App P-9 Ref.)*. Many keto diets are chock-full with inflammatory foods that are high in saturated fats (bacon, cheese, red meats, etc.). In this book I introduce the "anti-inflammatory diet with keto push." This is a keto diet that is based on anti-inflammatory foods to avoid the unhealthy options. It is difficult to balance carb intake and keep the fat content high. In the book I describe how you can balance healthy carbs and healthy fats to keep your net carb intake to less than 50 net grams per day. I refer to this modification of the typical keto diet as the AI-keto (eye-key-toe) diet. This is a healthier alternative to the "dirty keto" diet and is similar to the "clean *(App P-10 Ref.)* keto diet" except it is focused on anti-inflammatory food choices.

The book separates the anti-inflammatory diet and the AI-keto diet as they are different in their goals as well as their diet plans. Readers will have the option to choose which diet plan bests fits their goals. The book is heavily referenced, providing reliable sources for most of the information. There is an electronic app that can be accessed to link to websites for references, recommendations and AIF recipes. If you purchase access to the electronic app at the Google Play Store or the Apple App Store you will be able to access the links within the app. App links will be categorized as references (Ref.), recommendations (Rec.) or recipes for anti-inflammatory meals (AIF). References will include materials on related topics, publications or videos. Recommendations will include; food items or products to help you in your quest to get uninflamed. The AIF links will include recipes to meals, meal plans, etc. Any link with a + designation is rated as high value. You can access information about the app at the website www.toriumidiet.com *(App P-11 Ref.+)*.

Throughout the book the reader will note callouts for figures. All of the figures are located in the figure section at the end of the book.

Readers who obtain the electronic version of the book will have access to the app with interactive links in the e-book format.

References, recommendations and AIF recipes are easily accessible directly within the e-book.

This book will provide you with the principles of the anti-inflammatory diet and AI-keto diet, diet plans and actual recipes to help you get on track. This practical information will make it easier to get healthier, strengthen your immune system and improve your existing medical conditions. The book promotes a healthier lifestyle to improve your chances of surviving the Covid-19 pandemic or future pandemics.

Acknowledgments

I would like to acknowledge Patricia Stahl for organizing and copy editing the book. I also thank M. Eugene Tardy and Joe Boozell for checking the content and editing parts of the book.

I also would like to thank Bridget Gillespie and Karen Mitchell for their work on the illustrations for the book.

Introduction

During the late winter of 2019 and spring of 2020, the entire world's population began to experience a pandemic of epic proportions. The "novel coronavirus," also known as severe acute respiratory syndrome coronavirus 2, or SARS-CoV-2 for short, infected millions of Americans and displayed a wide range in severity of disease, with many people showing no symptoms, yet others demonstrating severe symptoms—even death. Those under 30 years of age tended to have mild to no symptoms and were rarely admitted to the hospital, whereas many over 60 years of age showed severe symptoms. The presence or absence of comorbidities is one of the key indicators as to what clinical course people had experienced. Comorbidities are chronic diseases that Covid-19 patients may have had when they contracted the disease. **Some of the most impactful comorbidities affecting Covid-19 outcomes are hypertension, obesity, diabetes, cardiovascular disease, asthma or other lung disorders.**[7] Additionally, age is a major risk factor given that death rates reached 20% in patients over 80 years of age, with hardly any deaths of those less than 20 years of age.

During the period of opening up the economy in the summer of 2020, many states experienced spikes in cases, filling of hospital beds and some deaths. The deaths were less than in the initial presentation of the disease, yet worrisome to the medical officials. It is unclear whether the Covid-19 pandemic will reappear in the winter and spring of 2021. Numerous experts are predicting that many people will again become infected with the SARS-CoV-2 virus unless an effective vaccine becomes available. No amount of social distancing or mask use will completely protect you from this very contagious virus. And even if a vaccine is developed, many may still become infected because first generation vaccines tend not to provide complete immunity. Most first generation vaccines help to decrease the severity of the disease if you become infected by the virus. Those who survive after getting infected with the SARS-CoV-2 will tend to have greater immunity that those treated with the vaccine. There is no guarantee that those infected in 2020 will not become reinfected in 2021. Considering the threat of the SARS-CoV-2 virus, we must think of ways to protect ourselves from suffering a poor outcome if we become infected.

If we look at the factors that influence potentially poor outcomes after contracting Covid-19, the one factor that we cannot control is our age. However, we have some control over the number of comorbidities that we have. Hypertension, obesity, adult onset diabetes and asthma are comorbidities that we can control to some extent. Heart disease and chronic lung diseases are less influenced by what we do on a daily basis. If we make significant lifestyle changes and modify our diets, we can decrease our blood pressure, lose significant amounts of weight, slim our waistline and even control our tendencies toward suffering an asthma attack. It is time for us to take personal responsibility for our general health by exercising and taking control over what we eat and drink.

There are many types of diets out there that are based on different underlying principles. There are plant-based diets, the Mediterranean diet, the Okinawa diet, the Paleo diet, low-carb diets, ketogenic diet, intermittent fasting diets, etc. This can be very confusing. My preference is the anti-inflammatory diet for several important reasons. First of all, it has similar characteristics of several other well-studied diets such as the Mediterranean diet, plant-based diets and the Okinawa diet. **The anti-inflammatory diet is based on eliminating or at least minimizing intake of inflammatory foods and trying to eat and drink either neutral or anti-inflammatory foods.** The diet requires a clear understanding of what is inflammatory and what is not, which I will explain in detail. It also involves incorporating anti-inflammatory supplements into your diet. Exercise is an important component to maximize the total body effect, as well. I will also discuss how you can incorporate a keto push into your diet to trim your waistline and help lose weight.

The anti-inflammatory diet defines a lifestyle that requires discipline and focus to implement. The only other means of protecting yourself from contracting a bad bout of Covid-19 is to isolate yourself. It has become apparent that is not a great option for an extended period of time as we know this can lead to loneliness, depression, alcohol abuse, drug abuse and even spousal abuse *(App 0-1 Ref.)*.[8] Other than isolating yourself, washing your hands frequently and wearing a mask, there are not a lot of other protective measures that you can take. However, you can change your lifestyle to protect yourself from a poor Covid-19 outcome should you contract it. You will benefit in many other ways as well. You may experience a definitive improvement in your overall health status, including significant weight loss, improved heart health, improved skin, less back and joint pain, improved self-esteem, better mood and a potentially longer lifespan.

The nasal passages are the most common pathway for entry of the SARS-CoV-2 virus. As a facial plastic surgeon trained in otolaryngology (ENT) who specializes in aesthetic and functional nasal surgery, I see the impact of inflammation on my patients' noses and sinuses. I also notice the impact of inflammation on my patients as they recover from nasal surgery. Many patients suffer from clinical symptoms related to their nasal function that compromise their quality of life. These symptoms could range from a stuffy runny nose to chronic recurrent sinus infections. Many of these patients take a multitude of medications to allay these symptoms. Medical care costs related to nasal and sinus disease are in excess of $60 billion every year[9]

Medications are prescribed and many surgeries are performed to alleviate the nasal and sinus symptoms. Unfortunately, these clinical interventions are all used to treat the symptoms and not the underlying cause.

Most things that we eat and drink will affect the inflammation in our bodies. What does this mean? Your immune system helps to control how your body responds to allergens and other environmental insults. When you get chilled, you may sneeze. This is more of a vasomotor response that is not related to inflammation. However, if you are allergic and are exposed to pollen, you may sneeze as well. You may also get very stuffy and have to blow your nose. This response is your body's immune system reacting to the pollen, and how vigorously you respond to the pollen depends on many factors.

With that said, the degree of inflammation in your body influences your degree of response. If you are inflamed, your response may be more pronounced. If your body's inflammation is lower, your response may be reduced to the point that you don't notice it. This may explain why you sometimes respond to allergens, but other times don't.

So what is inflammation? There are acute and chronic forms of inflammation. Acute inflammation occurs when you are fighting an infection or recovering from an injury. Whole body chronic inflammation can result from eating poorly, stress, exposure to toxins, etc. In response, your body circulates white blood cells and chemical messengers. The white blood cells and abdominal fat cells (visceral fat) can release damaging hormones such as tumor necrosis factor, IL-6 and free radicals. These hormones can damage your organs, obstruct your blood vessels, damage your brain and even cause cancer.

Inflammation also affects many other bodily functions. Some examples: your back and joints may be sore after activities if you are inflamed. Your back may hurt more when you wake up in the morning when you are inflamed. Your skin may be more acne prone with increased redness when you are inflamed. Believe it or not, your body's inflammation is linked to heart disease, arthritis, rosacea and, yes, your nose and sinuses. Your body's inflammation may also affect your vulnerability to contracting Covid-19 and the severity of your infection. In fact, research had shown that treatment with a steroid, dexamethasone, demonstrated promising results with severe cases of Covid-19. In many of these cases, there was an accentuated immune response to the virus. This hyperactive immune response worked against the patient, fueling a more severe response in the lungs, frequently resulting in acute respiratory distress syndrome (ARDS) and potential death. Patients treated with dexamethasone showed a 20% lower risk of dying from Covid-19 *(App 0-1 Ref.)*. The theme here. Inflammation is bad for your body and your general well-being.

So how do you control your body's inflammation? You actually have more control than you may think. Most things that you eat or drink will affect your body's inflammation, and your diet is closely linked to how your body functions and how you feel. Some foods are inflammatory and increase your body's inflammation. Other foods are anti-inflammatory and decrease your body's inflammation. Many things are neutral, so they do not affect you either way. Additionally, many foods will affect people differently, with some people becoming inflamed when they eat inflammatory foods and others not affected to the same degree. Think of the food you eat and drink as fuel. If you eat and drink bad fuel (inflammatory foods) you will become inflamed. If you eat and drink good fuel (anti-inflammatory foods) you will become less inflamed.

The first thing that you will need to understand is how foods influence inflammation. Next you need to find out what foods and drinks are inflammatory or anti-inflammatory. In this book I will empower you to make your own educated decisions on what to eat on a daily basis. I will give you sufficient background information on how your body responds to food and drinks. I will also teach you how your body's immune system is influenced by what you eat. We can then go into some detail about what foods are inflammatory and what foods are anti-inflammatory. You will thus be empowered to help control your body's overall function and improve your quality of life. The overall goal here is to feel better and eliminate some of those comorbidities that can negatively impact your experience with SARS-CoV-2 or other future viruses.

I will start by explaining how your nose and sinuses work and how they are impacted by inflammation. As previously mentioned, SARS-CoV-2 likely enters your body via the nose and if your defenses are strong, perhaps your body can fight off some of those viral particles that are spread when someone near you with Covid-19 sneezes or coughs.

1 YOUR NOSE, SINUSES AND IMMUNE SYSTEM —THE FIRST LINE OF DEFENSE AGAINST COVID-19

The SARS-CoV-2 virus that causes Covid-19 has spike proteins on its surface that bind to cellular receptors in the human body. The virus needs the ACE2 receptor protein and the TMPRSS2 enzyme to actually enter cells. It just so happens that ciliated and mucus-producing goblet cells in the nose have a very high number of these receptors and are likely the primary route of infection for the SARS-CoV-2 virus *(App 1-1 Ref.)*.[10] (Figure 1) **All of the figures are in the figure section at the end of the book.**

Nose and sinuses

It is likely that the nose is the primary means for the SARS-CoV-2 virus to enter the body and infect us *(App 1-2 Ref.)*. The nose may also be one of the primary means for the virus to spread to others through secretions shed when we sneeze or even breathe normally. Interestingly, loss of smell (anosmia) in the absence of nasal obstruction is a key indicator of Covid-19. With the common cold you may get some decrease in smell and taste, but in combination with nasal obstruction. The loss of smell with no obstruction is unique to Covid-19 *(App 1-3 Ref.)*[11].

Your nose is composed of two channels that permit airflow to the back of your nose and then down past your vocal cords and into your lungs. The two airways or channels are divided by the nasal septum, which is a partition that separates both cavities. Your nasal cavity is lined with nasal epithelial cells with cilia that move debris. This is the lining that may bind to the SARS-CoV-2 virus and infect you. You also have sinuses in your head that are connected to your nasal cavities. Most humans have six sinuses that are paired. There are two frontal sinuses that are located in your forehead region, two ethmoid sinuses that are located behind your eyes and two maxillary sinuses that lie under your cheeks. (Figure 2) Your sinuses open into the nasal cavity through small openings called ostia. The ostia communicate with your nasal cavity and allow the sinuses to drain into your nose. Your sinuses are usually filled with air but can become filled with fluid.

Your nose and sinuses are closely connected and are lined with a reactive tissue layer called mucosa. As mentioned above, this mucosa is ciliated and has the ACE2 receptor protein. However, the mucosa in your nose and sinuses has more blood vessels, is very moist and actually can evaporate water very effectively to humidify the air that you breathe. To accomplish this, the blood vessels in the mucosa in your nose and sinuses have the capacity to become engorged with blood and make the mucosa swell or expand. When the mucosa becomes engorged with blood and swells you enhance your ability to humidify the air that passes through the nose and sinuses. You may also experience nasal blockage because the enlarged mucosa blocks your nasal airway. This may compromise your ability to breathe through your nose. If the mucosa swells you will also notice that your nose may drip and you may have more secretions. This is all part of your body's response to some allergens, environmental insults or just changes in local conditions (temperature, humidity, wind, etc.).

You also have structures called turbinates that are smaller bony projections along the side of the nasal cavity that actually partially block the nasal airway. There are inferior, middle and superior turbinates. (Figure 3) The turbinates are covered with mucosa and act to increase mucosal surface area to maximize humidification of the air that passes over the turbinates. The turbinates also act to create resistance to nasal airflow to help control airflow. Sometimes one can look into the nasal airway and it may appear that the airway is blocked by the turbinates. If the turbinates are removed, one may lose the feeling of airflow through the nose as the airway may be too large. Additionally, a person may not be able to adequately humidify the air that he or she breathes, making it uncomfortable to inhale. Some patients may actually develop "empty nose syndrome" from scarring and over-reduction of the inferior turbinates. These patients can experience pain, dryness, abnormal sensations in the nose or other symptoms. The turbinates are covered with ciliated mucosa, with the ACE2 receptors providing a large area for the SARS-CoV-2 virus to attach. As you can see the nose and sinuses are completely lined with the receptors to permit passage of the SARS-CoV-2 virus.

Sometimes the nasal septum is deviated and can block the nasal airway or compromise nasal airflow. Correction of a deviated septum may require surgery: a "septoplasty" to straighten the nasal airway. However, if you are able to breathe well at times but get blocked at other times, this means you have "reversible nasal blockage." This means the fixed structures in your nose are not the primary cause of your nasal obstruction or that your obstruction is multifactorial. For some patients it's due to a deviated septum, while in others it's due to the fluctuations in swelling of the internal lining of the nose.

Reversible nasal blockage is usually due to swelling of the mucosal lining of the nose and can be triggered by nasal allergies or vasomotor reactive swelling. Vasomotor swelling is usually due to reactivity to environmental insults such as noxious inhalants (smoke, particulate matter, etc.) or exposure to hot and cold extremes. The response is to cause swelling of the mucosa and also to increase nasal drainage from the mucosa to keep the nasal airway moist. These responses are your body's normal response to changes in the inhaled air to protect you. Some patients have a more reactive airway to these environmental factors. With allergies, the mucosa in the nose swells and blocks the airway. This is not the case with Covid-19 and should not be confused with allergies. Reversible nasal blockage can also be caused by reaction to allergens. The response to allergens is less vasomotor and is triggered by a cascade of events once an allergen reaches the nasal mucosa.

Covid-19 and loss of taste or smell

Many patients who contracted the SARS-CoV-2 viral infection developed the symptom of loss of taste and/or smell. In a study of Covid-19 patients, smell was lost in 68% of patients, and loss of taste was noted in 71% of patients.[12] Most patients (74%) noted recovery of their taste and smell after the resolution of their viral infection. We are not sure of the etiology of the loss of taste and smell; however, it is likely due to either swelling or inflammation in the area of the olfactory neurons, as taste is closely linked to smell. Loss of smell is noted with many human viral strains, including other coronaviruses.[13] Study of the loss of smell with the SARS-CoV-2 virus suggested involvement of the olfactory neurons (smell nerves) or infection of the non-neural olfactory epithelial cells.[14] It is logical that the SARS-CoV-2 virus attacks the olfactory epithelium, which can rapidly regenerate and repair after the virus infection is over.

In either case, one of the routes of viral infection is likely via inhaling the virus. That is why we wear masks. This is also why social distancing is important to create a boundary where the virus is unable to reach our nasal cavity and cause infection. This is also why those who are infected or potentially infected should wear a mask to block viral particles if they should cough or sneeze. All of these measures will help prevent the spread of the virus during the next virus season.

The role of the immune system

The allergic reaction begins with your immune system. When you react to dust, pollen or mold, your immune system may overreact by producing antibodies that attack the allergens with a resultant reaction causing a runny nose, sneezing, watery or itchy eyes and other symptoms such as fatigue. In this case your immune system is working against you and causing your allergic symptoms. If you have allergies, you are not alone. Nearly 18 million adults in the United States have hay fever or allergic rhinitis *(App 1-5 Ref.)*. The Centers for Disease Control and Prevention notes that allergies are the sixth-leading cause of chronic illness in the U.S. and cost Americans more than $18 billion a year.

In most cases your immune system is helping to protect your body from infection due to bacteria, viruses and any other infectious organisms that try to invade your body. The immune system is composed of blood vessels and lymphatic vessels that carry lymphocytes to different parts of the body. The lymphoid organs are responsible for maturation of your immune system and the production and release of lymphocytes, which are a type of white blood cell in your body.

There are multiple lymphoid organs scattered throughout your body. The lymphoid organs include your adenoid glands and tonsils located in the back of your nasal passages and throat, respectively. (Figure 4) Your adenoid glands and tonsils are primarily functioning when you are young and tend to atrophy as you get older. Your appendix is another lymphoid organ that is a small tube-like organ that is connected to your large intestines. Some people have their appendix removed if it becomes infected. The lymphatic vessels are part of your lymphoid system and allow movement of lymphocytes throughout your body. Your bone marrow is an important part of the lymphoid system and is found in the core of the bones in your body. It is a softer, almost fatty type of tissue within the inner cavities of your bones. Some patients will undergo a bone marrow transplant to reestablish their immune system if it is destroyed with chemotherapy. Your lymph nodes are smaller lymphoid organs that are located throughout your body and are interconnected via the lymphatic system of vessels. Common sites for lymph nodes include your neck, underarms, groin and within your chest and abdomen. The paired thymus glands are located in the neck and are just in front of your trachea and behind your breast bone. Your spleen is in your abdominal cavity, is highly vascular and is located on the left side of your abdomen.

When you have an allergic reaction to an allergen, typically it is an overreaction of your body's immune system to a substance that would not cause an immune response in others. This overreaction is likely due to increased inflammation in your body that is linked to your immune system. Your immune system will produce immunoglobulin E (IgE) for each allergen that you respond to. Thus each IgE antibody is specific for a particular antigen. Ragweed will have one IgE antibody and mold will have another IgE antibody. The IgE antibodies will then attach to your body's mast cells and to basophils. (Figure 5) When you are exposed to the antigen again once the IgE is present in your body, it attaches to the IgE like two puzzle pieces fitting together. This signals mast cells to release the histamine and will cause the symptoms of an allergic reaction (runny nose, sneezing, watery eyes, etc.).

We really don't know what causes allergies.[15] There tends to be a hereditary connection as allergic adults typically have allergic children *(App 1-6 Ref.)*. However, there is no known direct genetic link at this point in time. One thing is apparent—inflammation is related to allergies. If you become inflamed, your allergies will tend to worsen. Therefore, decreasing your body's inflammation will tend to improve your allergies and nasal symptoms. This is where the anti-inflammatory diet can help with your nasal allergies.

If the nasal mucosa swells the airway can become blocked, creating nasal obstruction. Additionally, the ostia to the sinuses can become blocked resulting in trapping of fluid in the sinuses. Once trapped the sinuses may become infected, creating facial pain and fullness. Patients will frequently experience fever, feeling of lethargy and lacking in energy, purulent drainage from the nose and nasal obstruction. Drainage of the sinuses is critical to clearing the infection. This can be accomplished by decreasing the mucosal inflammation through nasal irrigation and medications to help shrink the mucosa. Once the mucosa shrinks the ostia open and the sinus contents will drain into the nasal cavity allowing the sinuses to recover.

The nasal mucosal response to the allergens is accentuated in the inflamed patient. In such cases your response to these allergens can be dampened if your immune system is modulated down to be less reactive. This gets back to decreasing your body's total inflammation. If you are less inflamed, you will tend to have less in the way of nasal symptoms. Some patients will constantly complain of nasal drainage and nasal stuffiness. Patients will frequently cite a specific day or time when their nasal symptoms were particularly bad. I will frequently ask patient's what they ate the night before they had their bad day or what they were eating during the time of their bad symptoms. The patient can frequently associate this time or day to inflammatory food intake. They may have had a pizza, dessert or drank some beer or wine the night before. When people travel they will frequently eat poorly because they're not at home and cooking for themselves. In this setting they may be eating out and not adhering to their normal diet. Their nasal symptoms may be much worse and then stabilize again once they are back home. Many people will end up getting sick or developing a sinus infection when they travel. This could be due to a combination of inflammatory foods, not sleeping well and exposure to more viruses and pathogens such as the SARS-CoV-2 virus. This is a good reason to really try to control your diet when you travel.

Many people will take multiple medications to help control their nasal symptoms. Common medications include Sudafed, Claritin and Zyrtec. Common nasal steroid sprays include Flonase, Nasonex and Nasacort. These medications act in different ways. Some are decongestants, antihistamines or nasal steroids. These medications all act to treat the symptoms of nasal allergies. I have seen many of my patients completely eliminate their use of allergy medications if they adhere to the anti-inflammatory diet. This is a tremendous feat for many of them as these medications can have annoying side effects and are costly. The objective is to prevent the inflammation in your body that can trigger the response to environmental allergens. This general decrease in your body's inflammation will provide many benefits—including decreasing your allergic symptoms.

CHAPTER 1: Your Nose, Sinuses and Immune System—The First Line of Defense Against Covid-19

Whether or not you contract Covid-19 may depend to some degree on the strength of your immune system and how well it can fight off an infectious agent such as a virus. Your immune system can produce infection-fighting cells such as white blood cells that can neutralize viruses. However, viruses such as SARS-CoV-2 can proliferate by invading cells in your body and taking over the cell in a way to allow it to replicate and make more viruses to spread further. Your body has special disease-fighting cells that can identify virally infected cells and destroy them with cytokines and other substances that can kill infected cells. Your body can also produce antibodies that can attach to the viruses directly neutralizing them. However, this requires antibodies to be formed by your immune system, which can take a bit longer and may help in a second exposure to the virus.

Bottom line: if you have a strong immune system you may be able to fight off the virus after exposure and not suffer the symptoms of the disease (cough, fever, loss of smell, body aches, etc.). This may be why many people who were exposed to SARS-CoV-2 never even presented with symptoms. If someone who has Covid-19 sneezes in your presence and you inhale the virus, the viral particles will have to attach to cells in your body to replicate and may cause symptoms. The incubation period is the time elapsed after you are exposed to the virus and when you first have symptoms. With Covid-19 this period can extend to 14 days with a median of four to five days. During the incubation period, the virus may be replicating and spreading throughout your body, ultimately reaching a threshold necessary for you to develop symptoms. Having a strong innate immune response during the incubation period can prevent the infection from taking hold, reduce the actual quantity of virus in the body, and prevent it from getting to the lungs. This is likely the scenario with people under the age of 18 or adults who go symptom free. Their immune response is such that the initial viral load of the SARS-CoV-2 virus is smaller due to the efficiency of their innate immune system and the rapid clearance of the virus upon exposure.

Eating inflammatory foods can worsen the comorbidities that make you more prone to a poor outcome if you contract Covid-19. Inflammation may also make your immune system less capable of fighting off the SARS-CoV-2 virus if it enters your body through your nose. Your nose is a key player in the Covid-19 battle and is one of the reasons I have discussed its anatomy and physiology. It makes sense to keep your nose covered with a mask, keep your distance from others if possible and keep your immune system as strong as possible.

2 THE GLYCEMIC INDEX AND INFLAMMATION

Diabetes is one of the most impactful comorbidities that can set you up for a bad outcome if you contract Covid-19, and it is important to do everything in your power to prevent or reverse it if possible. Diabetes also may have a tremendous impact on cardiovascular disease, kidney damage, nerve damage, vision, brain function and problems with blood flow to your extremities. There are three major types of diabetes; Type 1 diabetes, Type 2 diabetes and gestational diabetes. Type 1 diabetes is thought to be an autoimmune disorder where the body attacks the beta cells that produce insulin in the pancreas, leaving permanent damage resulting in reduction of insulin production *(App 2-1 Ref.)*.[16] Type 2 diabetes is typically preceded by prediabetes and indicates that you have higher than normal insulin levels in your blood. Prediabetics will have impaired glucose tolerance, which is higher than normal glucose levels in the blood after a meal. They will also have an impaired fasting glucose, which is a higher than normal glucose level in the blood prior to your first meal of the day. You may also have a hemoglobin A1c between 5.7 and 6.4 percent. Hemoglobin A1c, or glycated hemoglobin, is hemoglobin with a glucose molecule attached and the normal levels are between 4 and 5.6. The hemoglobin A1c tests the average amount of glucose in the blood over the last two to three months by measuring the percentage of glycated hemoglobin (A1c) in the blood.

Risk factors for prediabetes include age over 40, obesity or high body mass index (normal BMI is 18.5 to 24.9) over 40, or if your waistline measurement is over 40 inches for males or 35 inches for females. Prediabetes is reversible and with proper diet, exercise and medication you can potentially hold off progression to Type 2 diabetes *(App 2-2 Ref.)*. If you are presently prediabetic, you should strongly consider wholesale changes to your diet and exercise routine to prevent the onset of Type 2 diabetes. Type 2 diabetes sets you up for developing other chronic diseases such as heart disease and stroke. Gestational diabetes occurs due to insulin-blocking hormones during pregnancy. According to the CDC, more than 34 million Americans have diabetes with 90 to 95% of people having Type 2 diabetes *(App 2-2 Ref.)*. That's particularly troubling in the midst of this pandemic, as Type 2 diabetes is one of the most harmful comorbidities you can have should you contract Covid-19.

The causes of Type 2 diabetes are lifestyle and genetics. You have no control over your genetics, but you have near complete control over your lifestyle. Granted, you may have some limitations due to family, your occupation or other physical disabilities that may make a certain healthy lifestyle more difficult. Most of us, however, have enough control over our lifestyle to make good choices such as exercising and eating well. Eating to prevent prediabetes begins with avoiding foods that have a high-glycemic index (GI).

The glycemic index is a scale that is used to classify carbohydrate-rich foods based on how fast they are digested and how they impact blood sugar levels in a two- to three-hour window after intake. (Figure 6)[17] The GI measures how fast different foods raise blood sugar levels in comparison with the absorption of 50 grams of pure glucose that has a GI of 100. Only carbohydrates will have a GI and foods that have no carbohydrates such as chicken, fish, meats and eggs will not be assigned a GI. Foods that have a low GI will be digested slower and will have less of an impact on insulin levels. High-glycemic foods will be digested quickly and cause a more rapid elevation in blood insulin levels.

GI will vary according to the types of sugars in a carbohydrate, the structure of the starch in the food or how refined the food is. Different sugars have different GIs. For example, fructose is a monosaccharide, has a GI of 19 and is a fruit sugar found in fruit, honey, agave, and most root vegetables. With its lower GI, one would think that fructose is a reasonable choice for prediabetics if a sugar is needed. This is not the case as processed fructose is very detrimental and can cause insulin resistance, raise triglycerides and increase visceral fat in your midsection. Agave nectar is very high in fructose and similar to high fructose corn syrup—it is not a good choice as a sweetener. All sugars have a mixture of fructose and glucose. Table sugar is 50:50 fructose to glucose. High fructose corn syrup is 55:45 fructose to glucose. Agave nectar is 90% fructose. Fructose that is taken naturally when you eat fruit is perfectly fine to eat. Apples have about 7% fructose. Andrew Weil has promoted using maple syrup in his restaurants as a sweetener if used in moderation as it has a lower GI of 54 *(App 2-3. Ref.)*. Choosing the right sweetener is very confusing and should be researched carefully as new ones come out frequently. In either case you should minimize the use of any sweetener and try to limit your intake of sugars through the fruit that you eat. If you are looking to institute the anti-inflammatory diet with the keto push, then most fruits must be limited as well. We will discuss the keto push in Chapter 8.

In general it is a good idea to avoid foods or drinks that have a higher GI. Most simple carbohydrates and juices have a high GI. White bread, most pastas and white rice all have a higher GI (greater than 70). Foods such as sweet potatoes, couscous and wild rice are medium glycemic (between 56 and 69). Complex carbohydrates such as broccoli and most other vegetables, nuts, chickpeas, apples and lettuce are low glycemic (less than 55). A diabetic diet promotes low-glycemic foods and avoids high-glycemic foods. The high-glycemic foods will tend to increase blood sugar and require your pancreas to secrete insulin. Working your pancreas very hard over the long term will potentially set you up for developing Type 2 diabetes. **In general, it is always better to eat low-glycemic foods and avoid high-glycemic foods. Most high-glycemic foods also tend to be inflammatory.** There are exceptions such as the sweet potato and steel cut oatmeal, which are anti-inflammatory. Steel cut oatmeal is different from instant oatmeal as the latter is high glycemic and inflammatory. Most instant oatmeals are processed with added sugars and should be avoided.

CHAPTER 2: The Glycemic Index and Inflammation

Highly processed high-glycemic foods can be extremely damaging in multiple ways. Foods such as donuts, bagels and processed breakfast cereals are high glycemic and also have potentially harmful additives that can promote heart disease or atherosclerosis. Any sugary drink that is artificially sweetened is particularly inflammatory and also potentially harmful to your cardiac health. You should stick to water and electrolyte replacement supplements with no sugars added (App 2-4 Ref.).

Many foods increase in their GI based on how much you cook them. For instance, if you undercook steel cut oatmeal it will be less inflammatory with a lower GI. But if you overcook steel cut oatmeal (soft and mushy) you may convert it to a high-glycemic food that will be more inflammatory. If you overcook a sweet potato you will increase its GI and make it more inflammatory as well. If you eat pasta that is al dente (slightly hard), it will have a lower GI, trigger less insulin in the blood and will be less inflammatory. Overcooked pasta that is soft or mushy will have a higher GI, trigger a higher insulin blood level and will be more inflammatory. The ripeness of fruits will also vary their GI. For example, a riper banana may have a higher GI of 48 and a less ripe (greener) banana will have a lower GI of 30. If you eat a banana that is showing browning of the peel then you can expect it will be softer and mushier and solicit a greater increase in glucose if eaten. If you like apples, eat firmer apples and avoid those that are softer as they tend to have higher sugar content, and thus will have a higher GI.

If you are prediabetic or have a genetic predilection for developing Type 2 diabetes, it is imperative that you work on a healthy lifestyle. Keys to preventing the onset of Type 2 diabetes include managing your weight and keeping your BMI in the normal ranges. If you are overweight, it is important to lower your BMI and decrease your abdominal girth. One of the best ways to decrease your waistline is to avoid eating moderate- and high-glycemic foods. The anti-inflammatory diet with the keto push is also a very effective means of decreasing the size of your waistline (discussed in Chapter 8). You should focus on eating complex carbohydrates, proteins and healthy fats. You must also exercise regularly to avoid becoming prediabetic. You should try to exercise every day and at minimum walk and climb stairs whenever possible. Try to stick to low-impact exercise such as swimming, biking and walking. Limit any processed foods and avoid fried foods and desserts. Eat anti-inflammatory and organic foods. Limit your alcohol intake as alcoholic beverages are simple sugars and will increase your blood sugar levels. Smoking cigarettes makes you twice as likely to develop Type 2 diabetes versus someone who doesn't smoke *(App 2-5 Ref.)*.

If you choose to eat high-glycemic foods (pasta, rice, bread, etc.), combine these with fat and acid in order to slow the rate at which the high-glycemic food is absorbed.[18] For instance, eating avocado, olive oil or nuts with a starch or sugar will tend to slow the rate the starch or sugar is absorbed. Adding an acid such as vinegar (balsamic vinegar, apple cider vinegar, etc.), lemon juice or lime juice will also slow the rate at which the starch or sugar is absorbed. The ideal combination is to eat a salad with olive oil and balsamic vinegar dressing with your meals to slow the absorption of any moderate- to high-glycemic meal choices. Add some slices of avocado to your salad to top off your meal.

One of the key issues when dealing with the prediabetic state is that your makeup may be influenced by cravings for high-glycemic foods. For many, this can be a difficult problem to overcome. My recommendation is to try to gradually shift into a low-glycemic diet by picking days of the week that you would consider eating some of your favorite high-glycemic foods. You may also find that on those days you feel much worse, with more back pain, joint pain and increased nasal symptoms. When you note these differences, it may make it easier to completely make the transition and get to a healthier state with fewer comorbidities, a less inflamed body and, as a result, a better chance of staving off Covid-19.

3 ANTI-INFLAMMATORY FOODS—THE KEY TO MANAGING YOUR BODY'S INFLAMMATION

Your body needs fuel to function properly. Everything you eat and drink is the fuel that allows you to go about your daily activities. Managing your body's inflammation requires that you carefully consider everything you eat and drink. It really comes down to making good choices. If you start your day with a cup of coffee you may be increasing your body's inflammation, depending on what you add to your coffee. If you drink black coffee you are likely neutral as coffee itself is not inflammatory. If you add cream and sugar to your coffee you are adding inflammatory items that can increase your body's inflammation. From this point on I will refer to food items as either pro-inflammatory (PIF), anti-inflammatory (AIF) or neutrally inflammatory (NIF).

Breakfast

It is important to start the day with a good meal. If you have a bagel with your coffee, you are adding another PIF that can increase your body's inflammation. Breakfast can be the toughest meal of the day due to schedules and our need to get out of the house and on the road to go to work. It's helpful to plan your AIFs ahead of time. Eggs are a good source of protein and can be cooked in advance as a hard-boiled egg and then refrigerated to eat on the go. If you would like to keep your cholesterol low, you can eat the whites and discard the egg yolks. Eggs are different based on how the hens were managed. Eggs that are high in omega-3 fatty acids are anti-inflammatory. Generally, any food that is high in omega-3 fatty acids is anti-inflammatory. Foods that are high in omega-6 fatty acids tend to be pro-inflammatory. Eggs that are high in omega-3 fatty acids are hatched from free-range hens. If the hens are fed corn products, then the eggs are likely higher in omega-6 fatty acids. In most instances, any animal food source that is fed corn is likely inflammatory.

Another option is to have a protein shake in the morning. It is relatively easy and quick to make and you can drink it while on the road or while working out. Consider a shake that consists of decaffeinated green tea, egg white protein, ground flax seed, chia seeds and frozen blueberries. Place up to 500 milliliters (about 17 ounces) of the decaf green tea, a large scoop of egg white protein powder, a large scoop of ground flax seed, tablespoon of ground chia seeds and 1.5 to 2 cups of frozen blueberries. You can downsize these proportions based on how much shake you would like. You can add other fruit such as strawberries or blackberries but should avoid bananas as they tend to be pro-inflammatory. You can use frozen organic blueberries that are relatively easy to find. Mix the ingredients with a blender and you have a refreshing, anti-inflammatory protein shake.

Ground flax seed is high in omega-3 fatty acids, dietary fiber and plant protein (four grams of protein in two tablespoons). Flax seed also will lower blood pressure, reduce arteriosclerosis, lower LDL cholesterol and prevent stroke. Flax seed has also been shown to decrease risk of prostate, breast and colon cancer *(App 3-1 Ref.)*. Mucilage, the primary soluble fiber in flax seed, combines with water to form a gel-like consistency that slows the emptying of the stomach. This leads to a feeling of fullness and can lead to a reduction in total caloric intake. A review of 45 studies on flax seed showed that the consumption of 30 grams a day (about two tablespoons) resulted in reductions in both body weight and waist measurement.[19] It is this gel-like filing of the stomach that allows the shake to make you feel satisfied until the next meal. You can also sprinkle flax seed in your steel cut oatmeal or add to your diet in the form of a flax seed and chickpea pasta.

If you are concerned about your testosterone levels, you should omit the ground flax seed from your shake as flax seed has the potential to lower testosterone levels *(App 3-2 Ref.)*. In place of the ground flax seed you can add ground chia seeds.

Chia seeds are loaded with anti-inflammatory agents and provide protein with few calories. One ounce of chia seeds has 11 grams of fiber, four grams of protein and five grams of omega-3s with only 137 calories. Calorie for calorie, chia seeds provide a tremendous source of nutrients with few added calories. The addition of chia seeds to the diet has shown to produce a reduction in weight through its soluble fiber called glucomannan.[20] You can add whatever you want to your shake, but if you want to lose weight and trim your waistline you must consider calories and the filling effect.

There are many protein options to choose from. If you have a dairy intolerance, you may want to consider and an egg white protein *(App 3-3 Rec.)*. Some soy proteins can be problematic because of reported health risks. Soy protein supplements may contain soy protein isolates. These can cause thyroid problems as well as other issues.[21] Choose an egg white protein that is a basic protein source with few additives *(App 3-4 Rec.)*. Another protein option is hemp seed, which is a plant-based protein and comes from hulled hemp seeds *(App 3-5 Rec.)*. Hemp seeds are also anti-inflammatory and deliver omega-3 and omega-6 fatty acids with a favorable omega-3 to omega-6 ratio of 3:1.

Another option for protein is almond milk, which has some anti-inflammatory properties *(App 3-6 AIF)*. Whey protein, mentioned above, is a popular choice but isn't without controversy. About 20% of cow's milk protein is whey. During the cheese-making process, casein coagulates into curd and settles to the bottom, while whey remains in liquid form and is drained off. This protein is then dried and processed, resulting in whey protein. Whey protein is a dairy product, and most dairy products are inflammatory. Some would argue that whey protein has many benefits, including enhancing muscle development. Other potential benefits include lowering blood pressure, decreasing abdominal inflammation, improving insulin sensitivity and reducing colon cancer risk. The problems with whey protein include issues with a lactose or milk allergy, preservatives added to the protein mix, and presence of oxidized cholesterol.

Many people use orange juice or other fruit juices in their shakes. You may want to consider changing to green tea to decrease the sugar content and gain the anti-inflammatory benefits of the green tea. If you would like to avoid caffeine you can use decaffeinated green tea to limit caffeine intake *(App 3-7 Rec.)*.

Consuming shakes for meals is a great way to lose weight. Many weight loss programs promote and incorporate shakes into their diet plans. The shakes can be fashioned to fill you up yet not expand your stomach. One of the best ways to shrink your stomach is to stop stretching it out. If you have a shake for some of your meals, the liquid will help shrink your stomach. If you have a smaller stomach, you will feel full quicker and may encourage you to eat less. You will have to avoid stretching your stomach during your other meals as well to really get the effect. You can mix up the contents of your shakes to provide variety and different flavors.

There are many options for ingredients to add to your shake. You may add avocado, which is anti-inflammatory and provides good fats. Avocado is high in calories, but is excellent for the person seeking to go on the keto push. Avocado also adds body to your shake. Many like to add bananas to their shake. Bananas provide a nice flavor and have some anti-inflammatory properties. However, they can be glycogenic, with a GI score of 48. Bananas should not be used while on the keto push.

Other things you can add to your shake include turmeric, ginger, spinach and kale. Turmeric has tremendous anti-inflammatory benefits. Ginger also has many healthy properties. Spinach and kale are very anti-inflammatory and will provide a nice supply of antioxidants. You can also add some matcha (Japanese green tea) to gain the benefit of the caffeine and antioxidants. By adding matcha you are adding ground tea leaves, which provides a higher level of antioxidant benefit and a longer-acting caffeine effect than coffee. Matcha will be covered in detail in Chapter 5.

Many people add yogurt to their shakes to give body and taste, but yogurt is a dairy product and is inflammatory. For the anti-inflammatory diet, it is better to avoid dairy in your diet and to keep your shakes as inflammation-free as possible.

Lunch

Lunch is a meal that can be planned ahead of time and prepared with anti-inflammatory ingredients. Salads are a good way to incorporate AIFs, but all salads are not created equal. Lunch salads can be very inflammatory based on what you add to them. You can use a baby lettuce mix (romaine, spinach, etc.). Romaine, kale and spinach are very healthy choices and are superior to iceberg lettuce, which has less nutritional value. Kale is extremely anti-inflammatory and contains many nutrients. Kale is actually a cruciferous vegetable that is rich in fiber, various amino acids, vitamins A, C, and K, iron, calcium and magnesium. The baby lettuces are easier to digest and tend to be more flavorful.

Chicken, salmon, garbanzo beans, almonds, walnuts, pistachios and hard-boiled eggs are all good protein sources on a salad. Tuna is also an option, but its mercury levels can be high. There are tuna options that are premeasured for heavy metals and are low in mercury *(App 3-8 Rec.)*. Monitoring mercury intake is very important to a healthy dieter who consumes a lot of fish. Many larger fish contain higher mercury levels and can cause mercury toxicity if too much is consumed. Smaller fish such as sardines are low in mercury. You should try to avoid eating larger fish, and if you put tuna on your salad, you should limit it to canned "light" tuna or a source of tuna that is measured low in mercury. Salmon is relatively low in mercury and is high in omega-3 fatty acids.

Cheese is a very popular topping for a salad. Unfortunately, most cheeses are pro-inflammatory. Adding small amounts of cheese to a salad is OK unless you are doing the keto push. If you want to adhere to strict AIF, you should avoid dairy products such as cheese. Cheeses are also higher in fat, and this can negatively affect your health. There are cheese substitutes that you can try. You will have to experiment to find one that's best for you. If you have trouble being satisfied with a salad for lunch, add avocado and nuts to the mix. All of these are AIF choices.

The key to an AIF salad is the dressing. Most dressings that contain dairy are likely pro-inflammatory. These would include thousand island, Catalina, ranch, Caesar, blue cheese, or any creamy dressing. Basically, most salad dressings are inflammatory. This is problematic because you think you are eating a healthy lunch but you may actually be eating an inflammatory salad. Avoid any dressing that has dairy or cheese in it. Also avoid any dressing with processed items such as high fructose corn syrup. High fructose corn syrup is very inflammatory and should be avoided. You can consider a balsamic vinegar and olive oil dressing. The dressing includes extra-virgin olive oil, balsamic vinegar, fresh garlic, salt, pepper, oregano, dill, parsley, thyme, garlic powder if fresh garlic is not available, basil and chili pepper. The mix is four to five parts olive oil to one part balsamic vinegar. Olive oil is anti-inflammatory and very healthy—it will be discussed in detail in the next chapter. Balsamic vinegar is anti-inflammatory as well and has many health benefits. You can also mix in some aged balsamic vinegar to add a little extra flavor. This dressing can be prepared ahead of time, is relatively easy to store and will keep for a week. The dressing is relatively low calorie and very healthy. By adding a fat in the form of olive oil and an acid in the form of balsamic vinegar, your body will more slowly digest high GI foods. If you are having some bread or pasta with your meal, the olive oil and vinegar will slow the absorption of the high-glycemic food choices, requiring less insulin release into your blood. This dampening of the insulin response to the higher glycemic foods is a great way to trick your body when you cheat on your diet or if you are on the keto push.

Garlic has potent anti-inflammatory properties.[22] You can put fresh garlic into your olive oil and vinegar salad dressing as well as over vegetables, meat, chicken and fish. It is a great replacement for dairy. Garlic will help with recovery after exercise and can decrease joint pain and symptoms of arthritis. Garlic has been shown to boost immunity and fight cancer cells and decrease the risk of heart disease[23]. If you are on a blood thinner medication, ask your physician if it is safe to use garlic in your diet as it can increase the medication's effect in a negative way.

Healthy sandwiches are another good lunch option. Consider almond butter or avocado on whole grain bread. The key is to choose your bread carefully. Always try to choose a whole grain option or a sprouted whole grain bread such Ezekiel bread. For the keto push you can use a keto-friendly option, which can have a low net carb of 2 per slice *(App 3-9 Rec.)*. Whole grain breads have a GI of around 50, and white bread has a GI of approximately 70. The grainier the bread, the lower the GI and the better it is for you. If you toast your bread on your sandwich or for breakfast, it will lower the glycemic index and decrease the insulin response. This simple alteration in the bread option can significantly change your body's response to the bread portion of your meal.[24]

Your protein choices could be sliced turkey, skinless chicken breast or a meat of your choosing. It is preferable to avoid red meats or processed meats as they tend to be pro-inflammatory. Most red or processed meat products contain saturated fats, and diets rich in this type of fat tend to promote inflammation. Cooked meats also contain advanced glycation end-products that have pro-inflammatory properties. **Avoiding red and processed meats in general will promote an anti-inflammatory diet.** If you choose sliced turkey, the less processing the better. Some of the smoked turkey options are processed. The best options are turkey slices carved from a turkey breast. You may have this option available at your deli counter. Different brands are noted for their degree of processing, and you can make good choices based on your research *(App 3-10 Rec.)*. You can cook a turkey or turkey breast and then portion the meat for sandwiches during the week.

Mayo versus mustard? Mayonnaise at a minimum contains egg yolk and some oils. It is higher in saturated fats and is inflammatory. Light mayonnaise may be better but is still higher in saturated fat than mustard. Most mayonnaise has some preservatives and other additives, making it a less-than-ideal option for a sandwich spread. Most deli mustards (Dijon or honey mustard) are composed of seeds of the mustard plant and some spices. The mustards in general are neutral and tend not to be inflammatory. The mustards are preferred over mayo in most instances. Just make sure there is no added sugar to the mustard. You should always check the labels when you purchase dressings or mustards and inspect for sugar content. You could replace a sandwich spread with an anti-inflammatory avocado spread or turmeric hummus *(App 3-11 AIF)*. You can add some romaine lettuce or other lettuce to add a juicy touch to your sandwich. Tomatoes are nightshade foods and are inflammatory. You could add onions, pickles, olives or lettuce instead. Other nightshade foods are eggplant and potatoes. These should be avoided as they will increase inflammation.

Soups can be very good, but many are high calorie and highly inflammatory. Any soup that is creamy likely has some type of dairy product in it, which makes it inflammatory. Any chowder or bisque has a creamy base. New England clam chowder and seafood (lobster) bisque are good examples of inflammatory soup options. You may think that broccoli cheddar soup is good for you because it has broccoli in it. On the contrary, this soup is high in calories and is inflammatory. Potato soups will be high calorie with a lot of carbohydrates and are likely inflammatory. Chili preparations have a mixed picture. Chili peppers contain capsaicinoids, which are anti-inflammatory, but chili is typically tomato-based. For this reason, many people will experience an increase in their nasal symptoms after they eat chili. If you can make a soup out of sweet potatoes or vegetables with no dairy, these may be good options.

Unfortunately, to enjoy an anti-inflammatory soup you may have to make it yourself. Most premade soups have some inflammatory ingredients that add flavor. If you make your own soup you can add things that you like and know are not inflammatory *(App 3-12 AIF)*. You can start with a chicken broth base or vegetable broth base and then add whatever you like that fits the AIF list of foods. You can take some cooked chicken or turkey and remove most of the meat and simmer the bones on low heat for a couple of hours. Remove the fat off of the broth after it cools for a bit. Take the broth and use this as the base for your soup. You can add broccoli, carrots, celery, sweet potato, onion, parsley, garlic, ginger, olive oil, apple cider vinegar, red pepper and ground turmeric. Cook the vegetables until they are soft. Then add shredded chicken or turkey. The meat should be added at the end as it is already cooked. This type of soup is very healthy and tasty and relatively low calorie. You can add salt and pepper for taste. You can refrigerate or freeze whatever you do not eat and have it at a later date.

Snacks

In the afternoon, many people may need a small snack to hold them over until dinner. This is where many people deviate from the AIF diet plan. Snacks such as potato chips, pretzels, candy bars and most protein bars are problematic. Good snacks include almonds, walnuts, pistachios and peanuts. The problem with nuts is that they tend to be high in calories, and once you start eating nuts, it's easy to eat too many. A good habit is to limit your intake to less than 10 almonds or a tablespoon of the other nuts. Other good snacks include carrots or vegetables with hummus made from garbanzo beans or edamame. Do not eat the hummus with chips, crackers or other carbohydrates. More quality options are baked kale, sweet potato chips, apple chips and baked carrot fries.

If you would like to eat a protein bar, there are a few that are less inflammatory. Because this changes constantly I have listed these on the app entry on AIF energy bars *(App 3-13 Rec.)*. For the most part, energy bars contain a lot of sugar, which is inflammatory. Look for energy bars that have no added sugar, have less than 20 grams of carbohydrates and less than 20 grams of sugar (not refined). Most of these energy bars get their sugar from fruits. Avoid chocolate bars or bars with preservatives. Another option is a celery stick with a tablespoon of almond butter on it. Try to avoid peanut butter as it tends to have added sugar or high fructose corn syrup added unless it is natural. Baby carrots with hummus are a great snack as well. Keep a hard-boiled egg in the refrigerator and pop one or two for a snack.

Dinner

Dinner is the one meal where we tend to splurge and stray from the anti-inflammatory choices. The way to plan dinner is to look at having a salad, complex carbohydrate and protein. The salad can be a baby lettuce mix with a balsamic vinegar and olive oil combo as discussed earlier. A great dinner option is to have a dinner salad. Dinner salads can include a lot of lettuce, a fist-size piece of protein and some nuts or avocado. You can use primarily romaine, kale and spinach. You can add a protein such as chicken, turkey, tuna, beans or nuts. Avoid adding too many beans or nuts to keep the caloric total down. You can add carrots, artichoke hearts, celery and/or asparagus. If you add avocado, you should limit it to less than one half of an avocado unless you are looking to add calories or fat to fill you up. Adding avocado to any meal is a good way to add fats that will satisfy your appetite very effectively, and avocado is frequently used with the keto push. Remember that the dressing is key. Avoid any of the inflammatory options with dairy or sugars and use abundant olive oil.

Choosing the right complex carbohydrate is also crucial. In most instances, this will be a vegetable of some sort. It is always a good idea to make the vegetable the primary part of the dinner. This is a shift from the past as most people plan around the protein or the starch. In the anti-inflammatory diet we eliminate the starch and replace it with a larger portion of the complex carbohydrate (vegetable). By making this shift to a larger portion of the complex carbohydrate we can decrease total caloric intake and increase the anti-inflammatory portion of the meal. In essence you are filling up on a lower-calorie food item. In order to accomplish this you will have to prepare vegetables in a fashion that make them more attractive and better tasting. Many vegetables are not great if simply steamed. However, most vegetables (broccoli, cauliflower, asparagus, green beans) become very appealing if they are baked or grilled with extra virgin olive oil and some salt and garlic.

If you are using the anti-inflammatory diet with keto push, the proportions change and the fats proportions are 55% to 60%, protein is 30% to 35% and complex carbohydrates is 5% to 10%. You can increase the complex carbs with the keto push if you add plenty of olive oil to the vegetables to increase the fat content.

The best options from an anti-inflammatory point of view are; broccoli, spinach, carrots, cauliflower and green beans. The key is how you cook these vegetables to make them more flavorful. For example, you can prepare broccoli placing the florets on a cookie sheet after dipping in olive oil. Too much olive oil will make the broccoli too oily and will add excess calories. Then sprinkle with salt. You can use garlic salt if you would like additional flavoring. Limit the salt if you have high blood pressure. You can use salt substitutes such as potassium salt replacement *(App 3-14 Rec.)*. Sea salt still has sodium and can increase blood pressure. Place the broccoli on a cookie sheet and place in the oven at 325 degrees. It is preferred to use a convection oven

CHAPTER 3: Anti-inflammatory Foods—The Key to Managing Your Body's Inflammation

setting if you have this feature. You can cook the broccoli on a barbecue grill at medium heat as well. Cook the broccoli until the florets are slightly crispy but not burned. This will take about 20 to 25 minutes—a bit quicker in the convection oven.

You can use a similar process with cauliflower and garbanzo beans. This combo is very tasty and anti-inflammatory. You can take the cauliflower florets, dip them in olive oil and place on a cookie sheet. Open a can of garbanzo beans and pour out the fluid, keeping the aluminum top attached. Add a teaspoon of olive oil to the can and shake it up for a minute. Then place the garbanzo beans on a cookie sheet and sprinkle with salt. You can also sprinkle with turmeric to add flavor, color and anti-inflammatory properties. Place in the oven on convection mode at 325 degrees. Cook until the florets are brown and the garbanzo beans are slightly crunchy. This will typically take around 30 minutes. The garbanzo beans are higher in calories and can be omitted if the caloric intake or carb count is to be limited. If you choose the cauliflower with garbanzo bean combination, you could make this 70% to 80% of your meal and just add a small piece of chicken, fish or meat. The garbanzo beans provide the necessary protein if you choose to leave out a meat item.

A similar method can be used to prepare kale chips. Take some kale and clean it thoroughly, then break it up into chip-size pieces. Avoid using the stems. Sprinkle the kale pieces with olive oil and salt. Place the kale pieces on a cookie sheet and grill at 325 degrees until slightly crispy. You will have to monitor the kale closely because it can overcook quickly. A large amount of kale will be needed because the chips will shrink. This will typically take about 15 to 20 minutes to cook. Kale is one of the most highly anti-inflammatory foods that is readily available. Kale is more nutritious if eaten in its raw state. However, the grilled kale chips are tastier if you are allowed salt in your diet. The problem with the kale chips is that they go quickly.

Another great anti-inflammatory complex carbohydrate option is to grill green beans with salt and garlic. Choose the French green beans as they are longer and more tender. Break off the top and end, clean them and place on a cookie sheet. Sprinkle them with olive oil and salt. Garlic can be added for taste. Fresh crushed garlic is the best, but if it's not available, garlic salt can be used as a substitute. Grill at 350 degrees until the green beans are slightly crispy and browned. This will typically take about 30 minutes.

Sautéed spinach is a great anti-inflammatory option for a complex carbohydrate. In this case the spinach is cleaned and then sautéed with olive oil, garlic and salt. Spinach is highly anti-inflammatory and is a very good option for a complex carbohydrate. A sautéed vegetable mix with green peppers, red peppers, yellow peppers, onions, broccoli, Brussel sprouts, green beans, kale and spinach is excellent. These can be combined and sautéed in a pan with olive oil, salt, pepper and garlic. Cook the Brussel sprouts, broccoli, green beans and cauliflower first and follow with the peppers. Finish with the onions, spinach and kale. These mixes take more work but make a great mixed vegetable option.

It would be a shame if I did not include artichokes on the list of top anti-inflammatory vegetables to include in your diet. **Artichokes have the highest levels of antioxidants and fiber content of any vegetable.**[25] Unfortunately, when we think of a vegetable we rarely think of the artichoke. In fact, many people have never had an artichoke and have no idea how to eat it or cook it. Don't think spinach and artichoke dip when you think artichoke. That is probably the worst option when it comes to consuming this valuable vegetable treat. The artichoke is actually the bud of a thistle, which is a flower. The leaves, or bracks, cover a fuzzy center called the choke.(Figure 7) Down in the core of the artichoke is the meaty core, called the heart. The heart is completely edible, easily contained and very tasty. A moderately sized artichoke will contain 10 grams of fiber *(App 3-15 Ref.)*. Artichokes are loaded with antioxidant-rich polyphenols as well as vitamins C and

K, potassium, magnesium and folate. The leaves of the artichoke should not be passed up to just eat the hearts. In fact, the meat on the leaves contains a tremendous amount of compounds found to lower cholesterol. The height of artichoke season is from March to May but can extend beyond that time in some areas of the world.

There are several different ways to prepare artichokes. Start by gently scrubbing the artichoke with cool water. On a cutting board, cut off the bottom stem and an inch off of the top of the artichoke. You could also cut off the tips of the leaves with scissors to get rid of the thorny projections. To cook them, you can steam moderately sized artichokes for 30 to 40 minutes. For larger artichokes, you may have to cook for close to one hour. To check if they are ready, push a fork into the base of the stem. If the fork will pass gently into the core, they are likely ready to eat. You can add some salt to the water. They can also be baked or grilled *(App 3-16 AIF)*.

My preferred way to roast artichokes is to start by cleaning the artichokes and cut off the bottom stems and an inch off of the top as noted above. Then create a cruciate shaped cut down the center of the top of the artichoke to make an opening. Squeeze a quarter of a lemon on the top of each artichoke and then rub the lemon on the cut end of the stem of the artichoke to minimize browning. Place one to three cloves of garlic into the center where the cut was made. Then add a tablespoon of extra virgin olive oil over the top and sprinkle half of a teaspoon of sea salt over the top as desired. Double wrap each artichoke in two layers of heavy duty aluminum foil to avoid drying out. Place upright in the oven or grill at 375 degrees Fahrenheit for approximately 45 minutes depending on the size of the artichoke. You can push a fork through the stem and if it is relatively soft they are ready to eat. Open the foil and serve. No dipping sauce is needed with this preparation.

To eat the artichokes, you can pick off the petals one by one and scrape the fleshy part off of the inside of the petals with your teeth. You will discard the tough green part of the petal. As you peel off the petals they will get softer and thinner. You can still eat the fleshy part with the softer smaller petals; there just is less to eat *(App 3-17 Ref.)*. You can dip the petals in a healthy dipping sauce made by gently heating olive oil with added crushed garlic and salt for taste. Once the petals are gone, you will have to remove the choke. If you eat this part you will surely choke on it. Once you reach the center of the artichoke, you can trim off the periphery to leave the soft center of the heart *(App 3-18 Ref. Video)*. Trimming the heart will take some practice to maximize the best part and minimize the ingestion of some of the more fibrous periphery of the heart. The heart is the best part of the artichoke and can be eaten by itself, with the dipping sauce, or added to salads, stews or soups. You can add artichoke hearts to a Mediterranean bowl with chickpeas, couscous, bulgur and avocado with turmeric and a protein such as chicken or tofu *(App 3-19 AIF)*. Because there are 4.2 grams of protein in an average size artichoke, you can use it as a protein source in a vegan diet. A tasty yet healthy way to eat the artichoke is to dip the components in an olive oil and garlic and salt dipping sauce. It's also nice that it takes some effort to pull the artichoke apart as it slows down the consumption of your meal.

The benefits of artichokes extend beyond their anti-inflammatory effects due to phytonutrient cynarin and flavonoid silymarin. Flavonoids such as apigen in artichokes have been shown to be active against pancreatic cancer cells.[26] Artichokes can also help with skin rejuvenation and act to decrease free radicals that can damage skin and cause skin cancers. Artichokes are plentiful in prebiotics and probiotics that positively impact the gastrointestinal flora composition *(App 3-20 Ref.)*. Artichokes have been used for years to help symptoms of irritable bowel syndrome (IBS).[27] The artichoke has also been known to improve symptoms of upset stomach, bloating and abdominal cramps. They also help with insulin sensitivity and are good for prediabetics. Because artichokes are gluten free, grain free, dairy free, low in fat and carbohydrates and are highly anti-inflammatory, they should be worked into your diet. Once you start to eat artichokes, they may become one of your favorite foods and definitely one of your favorite vegetables.

Should you use organic produce? A meta-analysis that looked at 343 peer reviewed publications showed that organic produce contained higher antioxidants than nonorganic produce.[28] Organic produce can be up to 40% more expensive than nonorganic produce. You will have to pick and choose when to go organic. The amount of pesticide that is sprayed on produce varies. The types that had the highest amount of sprayed pesticide were spinach and kale *(App 3-21 Ref.)*. So if you decide to buy spinach or kale I recommend that you buy organic. It is also preferable to go organic when you buy apples, strawberries, blueberries, grapes, peaches, nectarines and cherries *(App 3-22 Ref.)*. The accumulation of pesticides and other potentially harmful additives could promote cancer or other harmful diseases later in life.[29]

Choosing the protein for your dinner can be very difficult, with many variables determining the anti-inflammatory value. For instance, any protein source that is high in saturated fats is inflammatory.[30] Foods that tend to be higher in saturated fats include red meats, processed meats (sausages, hot dogs, bacon, etc.) and cheese. Meats can be higher in saturated fats based on how the animals are fed. For example, grass-fed beef contains much less saturated fat than grain-fed beef.[31] If you must have your red meat, select grass-fed beef. Most beef cattle are fed grain (corn) as a more concentrated form of feed so the animals will grow faster and add more marbling (saturated fat). These meats are more flavorful but are also more inflammatory. If marbled beef is a favorite food, just eat a very small portion about the size of a hockey puck and fill yourself up with olive oil sprinkled over broccoli, cauliflower, garbanzo beans or another vegetable or salad.

Chicken breasts without the skin are very good and low in saturated fats. Keeping the skin adds saturated fat and makes the meat inflammatory. If you are eating chicken wings, you are eating an inflammatory meat with lots of saturated fats. It may be chicken, but not all chicken options are anti-inflammatory. Organic, grass-fed, free-range chickens are higher in omega-3 fatty acids, making them more anti-inflammatory *(App 3-23 Ref.)*. Corn-fed chickens are primarily given ground corn and corn cobs to eat to make them grow faster. Grass-fed chickens tend to be smaller and grow slower. In general, grain-fed chickens are lower in omega-3 fatty acids and conjugated linoleic acid compared to free-range chickens. Feeding chicken corn creates an unfavorable ratio between omega-3 fatty acids and omega-6 fatty acids. Grass-fed chickens will tend to have a 1:2 to 1:4 ratio between omega-3 fatty acids to omega-6 fatty acids, whereas, corn-fed chickens will tend to have a 1:20 ratio between omega-3 fatty acids and omega-6 fatty acids. It tilts the scale to a much more unfavorable ratio, negating the potential positive effect of the omega-3 fatty acids *(App 3-24 Ref.)*. When choosing chicken for your protein, choose chicken breasts that are organic, grass-fed, free-range. If you do not want to spend the extra money, you can use chicken breasts with the skin on it and cook it with the skin on but take the skin off when you eat it. At least by taking off the skin you will be eliminating some of the omega-6 fatty acids.

A great way to cook chicken is to spatchcock it with the skin on it. Choose an organic, free-range, grass-fed whole young chicken. In this case, the chicken is split along its spine and spread across a cookie sheet with the skin facing up *(App 3-25 AIF)*. Place sliced lemons under the skin of the chicken. With the skin and inserted lemons on the chicken, rub olive oil over the surface of the chicken. Then sprinkle a generous amount of salt and thyme over the chicken. Cook the chicken at 325 degrees on convection mode for about an hour and a half until the skin of the chicken is browned. You can also cook a spatchcock chicken on the grill on low heat. When you eat the chicken you can remove the skin to decrease the saturated fats and keep the anti-inflammatory effect. Remember that the breasts are white meat and the thighs are dark meat. Chicken thighs have double the amount of fat than chicken breasts with seven grams of fat in three ounces of cooked chicken thighs versus three grams of fat in three ounces of cooked chicken breast. However, there is only one more gram of saturated fat in chicken thighs compared to chicken breasts so the differences are not harmful to you. You will essentially double the fat intake if you eat a chicken thigh with skin versus without the skin. You will always be better off if you eat a chicken breast rather than a thigh unless of course you are on the anti-inflammatory diet with keto push where you are trying to increase your fat intake.

There are obviously many other ways to cook chicken. You can grill chicken breasts using different seasoning options. You can simply apply some olive oil, salt, pepper and add a seasoning to spice up the meat. You can use salt, oregano, garlic, lemon, black pepper and marjoram *(App 3-26 AIF)*. You can purchase such a mixture from some spice companies *(App 3-27 Rec.)*. This chicken breast recipe is great for cooking on the grill. You should avoid barbecue sauces as they tend to be sweet with a lot of sugars such as high fructose corn syrup. Most barbecue sauces are also tomato based, making them inflammatory. This makes your nice lean chicken breast very inflammatory. A low-sugar barbecue sauce would be a good option *(App 3-28 AIF)*. In some of these options you can forgive the tomato base if the sugar content is relatively low.

Another great protein option is salmon. Salmon is hatched in fresh water, travels to salt water and then returns to fresh water to spawn. Salmon are anadromous as they hatch in fresh water, migrate to the ocean, then return to fresh water to reproduce. Salmon can be purchased in a lot of different forms. In most instances you will be purchasing farm-raised salmon. Typically, farm-raised salmon are fed corn products and corn byproducts high in omega-6 fatty acids. Wild salmon eat krill, smaller fish and algae, all rich sources of omega-3 fatty acids and antioxidants called astaxanthin. **Wild salmon are found to be anti-inflammatory and farm-raised salmon are inflammatory.** In Monica Reinagel's book *The Inflammation-Free Diet Plan: The Scientific Way to Lose Weight, Slow Aging, Prevent Disease, and Banish Pain* she created the Inflammation Factor (IF) rating scale. It rates three ounces of wild salmon as one of the most anti-inflammatory foods that you can eat and three ounces of farm-raised salmon as highly inflammatory.[32]. In her book, she uses an inflammation factor rating the three ounces of wild salmon with an IF factor of 518 (this is good), and three ounces of farm-raised salmon with an IF factor of -181. To give perspective, a half cup of chocolate ice cream has an IF rating of -127. A negative IF factor is pro-inflammatory. I believe Reinagel's IF rating resource is a good place to learn about which foods are anti-inflammatory, which are pro-inflammatory and which are neutral. Obviously you will want to try to eat the foods that are anti-inflammatory or neutral *(App 3-28 Ref.)*.

You should try to purchase wild caught salmon for your meals. However, wild caught salmon can cost three to four times more than farm-raised salmon *(App 3-29 Ref.)*. This can be a big issue for many people. Most salmon sold at restaurants will be farm-raised. If the menu says "wild" then it may be wild caught. If it does not say on the menu that is it "wild" then it is likely farm-raised. Farm-raised salmon is usually sourced from the Atlantic Ocean and then hatched, raised, and harvested in a controlled environment. Wild caught salmon is usually from the Pacific Ocean and is typically caught during the summer or late spring. If you see "Atlantic salmon," it is likely farm raised. If the salmon is Alaskan salmon it may be wild caught or farmed but is likely from Alaska.

Is it worth eating farm-raised salmon? Compared to wild salmon, farm-raised salmon is much higher in fat, containing slightly more omega-3s, much more omega-6 and three times the amount of saturated fat and many more calories. But eating farm-raised salmon is likely better than eating fatty red meat as it still has a relatively high amount of omega-3 fatty acids. The bigger problem with the farm-raised salmon is likely related to the organic pollutants such as polychlorinated biphenyls (PCBs). Conversely, wild salmon is higher in minerals, including potassium, zinc and iron and likely lower in PCBs. Wild salmon is going to give you the benefit of the omega-3 fatty acids, is anti-inflammatory and is lower in fat content.

Other fish sources can be broken down into salt water options and freshwater options. Salt water options include tuna, halibut, cod, grouper, king and Spanish mackerel. Most of these fish are wild caught. The issue with most of these fish is the mercury content and PCBs. Everyone who eats fish should be aware of the mercury content in larger fish. Mercury builds up over time as fish get larger due to eating a lot of smaller fish that contain mercury and PCBs. Larger fish such as tuna, swordfish, King and Spanish mackerel, grouper and sea bass can be very high in mercury. Mackerel is higher in mercury but is also one of the highest in omega-3 fatty acids. If you can find a smaller mackerel it may be a good option to broil in the oven as a source of omega-3 fatty acids. Sardines are high in omega-3 fatty acids and are a smaller fish with low mercury. Sardines can be used in a salad or eaten directly from the can. They can also be grilled and eaten as a protein source. Sardines can be used on a pizza made with a cauliflower crust, mushrooms, red peppers, onion, and soy cheese substitute *(App 3-30 AIF)*.

Medium-sized fish such as halibut, cod, mahi mahi and snapper have intermediate mercury levels *(App 3-31 Ref. +)*. These fish options can be grilled or sautéed with a complex carbohydrate. These fish should only be eaten occasionally to avoid increasing mercury levels.

You should only rarely eat the high mercury options and only in smaller quantities. This is particularly important in pregnancy as the mercury can damage the fetus. If you choose to eat sushi you can eat salmon safely. Some smaller tuna will have lower mercury. If you frequent a sushi restaurant that has multiple grades of tuna (super white, fatty tuna (toro), etc.) then the regular tuna (maguro) likely comes from a larger tuna and likely has higher mercury levels. If you go to a smaller local neighborhood sushi place that has maguro and no other tuna options then the sushi may be cut from a smaller fish and may have lower mercury levels. There are companies that sell tuna that is tested for mercury levels so you can be sure you are not ingesting excessive amounts of mercury *(App 3-32 Rec.)*.

A great healthy recipe is a stuffed red snapper cooked on the grill. It's essential to have fresh red snapper, though it can be hard to find unless you are on a southern coast of the U.S. or other warmer destinations. You can prepare the whole red snapper leaving the scales on. You should fill the cavity of the fish with a mixture of chopped red peppers, onions, crushed garlic, olive oil and seasonings (salt, pepper, etc.). If you would like a spicy kick, you can add some chopped jalapeño pepper. Jalapeño peppers are anti-inflammatory, and a medium-sized jalapeño has between .01 grams and six grams of capsaicin. Capsaicin is a vasodilator that is anti-inflammatory. It has been used for arthritis pain, nerve pain and even dermatological conditions *(App 3-33 Ref.)*.[33] The mixture is simmered down on low heat for 20 to 30 minutes. After placing the heated mixture in the cavity of the red snapper, you can place a tie around the fish or place in a fish basket to keep everything in place. Then place the whole fish on the grill on low to medium heat and grill for about 20 to 30 minutes or until the outside of the fish is crispy. You can serve the entire fish on the plate. The scales and skin will easily peel right off of the fish leaving the steaming tasty fish meat underneath the skin. The remainder of the mixture of pepper, onions etc.

can be used as a sauce over the fish to add the final kick to the dish.

Another option is to make a blackened mahi mahi on a hot plate. Take some fresh mahi mahi steaks and cover with a thin layer of olive oil. Add jerk fish seasoning over the fish fillets and place the fillets on a very hot grill plate to sear the surface of the fish *(App 3-34 Rec.)*. The outside should be cooked and the inside kept moist. This will usually take about five minutes per side.

Freshwater fish tend to be lower in mercury and lower in omega-3 fatty acids.[34] Freshwater fish do not eat krill, which is where the build-up of omega-3 fatty acids starts. Freshwater fish are still a good source of protein, but unfortunately are not as anti-inflammatory. Fish that are limited to fresh water that are good to eat include trout, bass, walleye, crappie, perch and eel. Tilapia is primarily a freshwater fish but is typically farmed and has all of the problems associated with farmed fish, such as lower omega-3 content and higher omega-6 content.

Other healthy proteins include legumes and chickpeas, nuts, eggs, tofu, tempeh, edamame, lentils and quinoa. Many of these protein sources can be used in a non-meat-based diet as a protein source. Some of these are more anti-inflammatory than others. Soybeans in general have anti-inflammatory properties and studies have shown that people who eat a large amount of soy proteins experience less inflammation.[35] It would be beneficial to incorporate soy milk, tofu and edamame (boiled soybeans) into your diet. There are many great ways to create a meal out of tofu. Tofu can be used as the primary protein source in a stir-fry with or without chicken. The key to a stir-fry is to keep the contents anti-inflammatory. These can include sliced vegetables such as yellow onions, carrots, peppers, mushrooms, celery, broccoli, asparagus, mung-bean sprouts and bamboo shoots. These can be sautéed in olive oil. The sauce used in the stir-fry is key. Most stir-fry sauces include a lot of sugar. This is obviously inflammatory. You can make up a sauce that contains ¼ cup of soy sauce, ½ cup of sake, one to two cloves of pressed garlic, one tablespoon of grated ginger root and one teaspoon of sesame oil. Most stir-fry recipes include sugar or a sweetener. My recommendation is to leave out the sugar and see if you like the taste. It may not be the same as other stir-fry dishes that you have tried in the past, but it will surely be anti-inflammatory. The sake adds a flavor that replaces the sugar. You can consider honey instead of sugar if you would like the sweeter flavoring *(App 3-35 AIF)*. After cooking the vegetables in the olive oil, you can add the tofu to heat it up then add the sauce and stir it in. Don't overcook to avoid making the vegetables too soft. Tofu can also be baked in the same sauce and served as a meat alternative. Try to avoid fried tofu.

Another great option for dinner or lunch is stew. Stews tend to have less liquid than soup and are heartier. To make a stew you can start with a chicken, turkey or beef stock. My preference is to use a chicken or turkey stock. The easiest method is to use a ready-made chicken or beef stock to start your stew. The best approach is to cook a chicken or turkey and remove the meat. If you would like a beef stew, use a lean cut of meat such as stew chuck. Then take the carcass after you remove the chicken or turkey meat, remove the fat, and place into a large stew pot and slow cook in water with some olive oil and salt and pepper. Let this simmer for a couple of hours, adding more liquid if needed. You can cook it down until you have the chicken or turkey flavor that you like. Then add vegetables such as carrots, broccoli, onions, green beans and whatever other vegetable you would like and simmer until they are soft. Finally, add the meat back to the stew and cook a bit longer but do not cook too long as the meat will dry out. Try to avoid using a tomato base or dairy products as they are inflammatory. You can also cook your stew in a slow cooker to thicken it up. One of the best things about a stew is that you can make a lot and then freeze the leftovers and simply microwave to heat up when you want to enjoy the meal.

Dessert

Is it reasonable to have dessert on an anti-inflammatory diet? Most desserts have sugar, and sugar is inflammatory. Therefore, it is not good to have a typical dessert such as ice cream, cake or pie. Fruit such as an apple is a good option to satisfy your sweet tooth. Granny Smith apples are considered the most anti-inflammatory and are the highest in fiber and polyphenols.[36] Granny Smith apples are also the lowest in sugar content. Red Delicious is another very good choice when it comes to anti- inflammatory benefits. Fuji apples are the highest in bioflavonoids (protects against heart disease and cancer). Gala apples are also high in bioflavonoids. Honeycrisp apples are high in fiber and are also a good choice. When you eat an apple you do not want to peel the skin as the skin carries much of the healthy benefits. It is also important to buy organic apples.

More dessert options include other fresh fruit such as strawberries, blueberries, cherries and oranges. Strawberries and blueberries contain the anti-inflammatory compound anthocyanins as well as fiber, vitamins and minerals. Cherries are high in anthocyanins and catechins. Because these fruits are not available year-round, you can purchase them frozen. These are relatively easy to find in your grocer's freezer section.

One of the problems we all have is that we simply eat too much. With the "super-sizing" or "value sizing" of the meal portions in the U.S., we tend to eat larger portions. The proper portion sizes should be about 1 1/2 to 2 1/2 cups of fruit, 2 1/2 to 3 1/2 cups of vegetables, 1/2 cups of whole grains and five to seven ounces of protein (meat, beans, and seafood) each day *(App 3-36 Ref.)*. These numbers are much lower than what we usually eat as Americans. There are several strategies to control your appetite and decrease your meal portion size *(App 3-37 Ref.)*. The objective is to shrink your stomach so you become satisfied quicker with less food and less caloric intake. Many people have bariatric (stomach reduction) surgery to make their stomachs smaller and then decrease their food intake. Ideally, we can create a similar effect without doing surgery. One strategy is to make sure that 20 to 30% of your total caloric intake is protein. This will make you feel more satisfied and also help to preserve your muscle mass. Complex carbohydrates such as vegetables should replace simple carbohydrates such as bread, pasta or rice. Adding olive oil to the vegetable will also satiate you. You can incorporate omega-3 fatty acids in fish and algae to your diet to decrease food intake as these foods increase the fullness hormone leptin.[37]

You can also consider exercising before you eat lunch or dinner.[38] **Exercise was shown to decrease brain activity in regions of the brain that are associated with the pleasures of eating food, reducing the motivation to consume food.** Exercise was also found to decrease levels of hormones such as acylated ghrelin and increasing levels of hormones such as peptide YY (PYY), pancreatic polypeptide (PP) and glucagon-like peptide 1 (GLP-1) that are known to suppress food intake.[39]

Eating a large green salad with olive oil and balsamic vinegar dressing at the beginning of your meal will help to curb your appetite as well. Try to avoid the higher-calorie salad dressings and stick to olive oil with balsamic vinegar. You should also eat solid calories instead of liquid calories. The simple act of chewing will promote the feeling of fullness by keeping the food stimulating the taste buds longer than a liquid would.[40] Additionally, liquids will not extend the stomach as would solid foods. This does not apply to water, as it has no calories and can help to stretch the stomach and decrease food intake. **If you drink two glasses of water before dinner, you will consume less food.**[41] You could gain a similar effect by eating a low-calorie soup before eating the remainder of your meal. A broth-based soup with some vegetables is ideal.

Food cravings are linked to your stress levels and the hormone cortisol. Cortisol levels increase with stress.[42] Many of us will fall back on eating comfort foods when we are stressed. This can be problematic in our busy lives as stress is a common daily experience. With the Covid-19 pandemic many people experienced increased stress, increased cortisol and resorted to increased food intake and perhaps even binge eating. The "quarantine 15" is similar to the "freshman 15" and refers to the weight that many people gained during the pandemic *(App 3-38 Ref.)*. Especially at the beginning, we were all social distancing, locked up in our homes and apartments and stressed out. Many turned to food to deal with the stress of the pandemic *(App 3-39 Ref.)*.

We must change our habits, and a good start would be to pivot away from binge eating to thoughtful eating. This means we have to develop a plan and follow it. Hopefully, we will not face the stresses of another pandemic anytime in the near future, and with stress levels back to our baseline levels we can better control our cortisol-influenced dietary habits. We can further lower our cortisol levels by increasing exercise, spending time with family and friends and focusing on an anti-inflammatory diet.

As you can see, with simple adjustments to your diet you can institute the anti-inflammatory diet. You will quickly note the improvement in your nasal and sinus symptoms, resolution of back and joint pain, improvement in your skin, decreased fat in your mid-section and weight loss. You will also just feel better. The major drawbacks include increased time requirements to prepare your meals, higher cost for the healthier food options and sacrificing some of your favorite foods. However, when you consider the negative health effects of continuing in an inflammatory state you will quickly recognize the long-term benefits of the anti-inflammatory diet.

4 OLIVE OIL AND ITS IMPORTANCE IN THE ANTI-INFLAMMATORY DIET

Olive oil and other healthy oils are important components of the anti-inflammatory diet. Oils are fats and are also important to a ketogenic diet. Extra-virgin olive oil contains more than 36 phenolic compounds. These phenolics have beneficial effects on inflammation, antioxidant status, antimicrobial activity and other biological markers of non-communicable disease.[43] One in particular is a non-steroidal anti-inflammatory agent, Oleocanthal. Oleocanthal inhibits cyclooxygenase (COX) enzymes and has powerful anti-inflammatory effects.[44] Oleocanthal acts on the same pathway as non-steroidal anti-inflammatory drug (NSAID) ibuprofen and acts to stop the inflammatory cascade by inhibiting both cyclooxygenase1 (COX-1) and cyclooxygenase2 (COX-2) inflammatory enzymes. Its effects are dose dependent and it has about 10% of the potency of the NSAID ibuprofen. The extra-virgin olive oil does not have the same side effects as the NSAIDS such as upset stomach, gastric ulcers, gastrointestinal bleeding, allergic reactions and liver or kidney problems. Extra-virgin olive oil is a natural anti-inflammatory that can be taken with every meal. A study of a range of Greek extra-virgin olive oils showed a concentration of oleocanthal ranging from 284 to 711 mg/kg.[45] And oleocanthal is unique only to olive oil and is not found in any other vegetable oils. Another phenolic compound in extra-virgin olive oil, oleuropein aglycone, inhibits the pro-inflammatory molecule TNFa. Hydroxytyrosol has been shown to reduce TNFa and interleukin1 beta with promising effects on other key pro-inflammatory molecules.

Extra-virgin olive oil is the primary source of dietary fat in the Mediterranean diet and has been recognized for years as a healthy dietary choice.[46] The incidence of chronic inflammatory diseases in Mediterranean populations is the lowest in the world, and life expectancy is among the highest.[47] Those living in Mediterranean countries consume 25 to 30 mL of oil per day as part of their diet, generally in cooking foods and as a salad dressing.[48]

One of the unique features of extra-virgin olive oil is the pungent flavor and irritation in the throat that one experiences when consuming the oil. Studies have shown that the oleocanthal is the compound causing this pungency and irritation.[49] Some have used the pungency and irritation to rate the quality of extra-virgin olive oils. In fact, the more bitter tasting a compound is rated, the more potent the anti-inflammatory, antioxidant, or antimicrobial actions of that compound may be.[50] Oleocanthal was found to inhibit COX-1 and COX-2 enzymes significantly more at equimolar concentrations.[51] They showed that oleocanthal (25 μM) inhibits 41% to 57% of COX activity in comparison to ibuprofen (25 μM) which inhibits 13 to 18% of COX activity. This data shows the powerful anti-inflammatory properties of extra-virgin olive oil and how it may impact those living on the Mediterranean diet.

There are numerous reported benefits of consuming extra-virgin olive oil beyond its anti-inflammatory properties. **The phenolic compounds in extra-virgin olive oil have been shown to inhibit the initiation and metastasis of many cancers.** This is demonstrated by the lower incidence of many types of cancer, including prostate, breast, colon and gastric cancer, in Mediterranean populations when compared to Western populations.[52,53] Oleocanthal is a COX-2 inhibitor and because COX-2 is implicated in the development of several cancers this may be the mechanism for the lower cancer incidence.

Extra-virgin olive oil is thought to be an important natural means of improving symptoms of degenerative joint diseases such as rheumatoid arthritis and osteoarthritis. When inflammation is increased, nitrous oxide levels go up and can negatively affect joints. Elevated nitrous oxide levels or related compounds are found in the joint fluid of patients with rheumatoid arthritis and osteoarthritis. Oleocanthal slows the production of byproducts of nitrous oxide in the joints and can improve symptoms and the progression of the disease.[54]

Olecanthal has also been shown to favorably influence neurodegenerative diseases such as Alzheimer's. Oleocanthal disrupts the phosphorylation of tau and the PHF6 peptide and B-amyloid peptides which can play a role in the progression of Alzheimer's.[55] [56] **Studies show up to a 40% decrease in Alzheimer's disease in populations consuming a Mediterranean-style diet.**[57] There is mounting evidence that oleocanthal, in conjunction with other phenolics, exerts a neuro-therapeutic potential that is reflected in the lower incidence of neurodegenerative disease in populations that regularly consume the extra-virgin olive oil.

Choosing a quality oil

How do you choose a quality olive oil? First of all, you must choose an extra-virgin olive oil. Extra-virgin olive oil is made from pure, cold-pressed olives and is the first product of the extraction process. Regular olive oil is a blend, including both cold-pressed and processed oils and has fewer anti-inflammatory properties. Cold-pressed oils that don't meet extra-virgin standards are typically refined to get rid of undesirable impurities, giving the oil a more uniform flavor and color. Extra-virgin olive oil is an unrefined oil and may have some sediment due to its minimal processing.

Try to use extra-virgin olive oil for your balsamic vinegar and olive oil dressing for salads, when applied to vegetables, or just to drink a teaspoon for the health benefit. Virgin olive oils are purely extracted from olives using mechanical means without chemicals but do not meet the same standards as extra-virgin olive oil. Pure olive oil (also simply called "olive oil" or "classic olive oil") is usually a blend of refined olive oil with less than 10% virgin olive oil. It tends to have little flavor and is best used for sautéing or cooking rather than for salads or for straight consumption.

There are some subtle differences in taste between Greek, Italian and Spanish olive oils. Spanish olive oil tends to have a golden yellow color with a fruity and nutty flavor. The Italian olive oil tends to be dark green and has an herbal aroma and a grassy flavor. It also typically has higher levels of cycloartenol that lowers cholesterol levels. Greek olive oil is usually green, packs a strong flavor and aroma, and contains more polyphenols than extra-virgin oils from Spain or Italy. The differences between Spanish, Greek, and Italian olive oils are not easily noticeable unless specifically labeled as from one of the countries. Typically a mix of three is sold in the same bottle. While the product may be labeled as Italian, it is actually a combination of oils from different countries, including Spain and Greece—but is packaged in Italy. Your selection of "pure" or "classic" olive oil options is not as critical as your selection of the extra-virgin olive oil.

Incorporating olive oil into your diet

There are many different ways to work olive oil into your diet. If you have a couple of salads during the day you can work in an olive oil and balsamic vinegar dressing. To prepare the dressing, you can add five parts extra-virgin olive oil, one part balsamic vinegar, one large clove of crushed fresh garlic, a pinch of salt and pepper, oregano, parsley, basil, thyme, dill and a touch of Cayenne pepper. This is a very healthy salad dressing that has plenty of antioxidant properties.

Balsamic vinegar contains polyphenols which are antioxidants that can protect the body from disease, defend against oxidative stress, and help with diabetes despite the fact that it contains sugars. [58] Ingestion of polyphenols enhances antioxidant protection and reduces cancer risk. Balsamic vinegar has an anti-glycemic effect, dampening the blood sugar spike after eating a meal.[59] The biologically active constituent of vinegar is acetic acid which inhibits the activity of several carbohydrate-digesting enzymes, including lactase, maltase and sucrase. When vinegar is present in the intestines, some sugars and simple carbohydrates temporarily pass through without being digested, having less impact on blood sugar levels. This essentially decreases the glycemic load of the meal, decreases the glucose in the blood and decreases the insulin response to the meal. This is important as a spike in blood sugar after eating increases demands on insulin production from the pancreas. Chronic high spikes in blood glucose set a person up for Type 2 diabetes. Diets with balsamic vinegar have shown to lower hemoglobin A1c, which measures the amount of glycated hemoglobin in the bloodstream over a 120-day period. A high percentage of glycated hemoglobin indicates problems with long-term blood sugar control. A1c results of 6.5% (48 mmol/mol) or greater indicate diabetes.

Balsamic vinegar also has an effect of making you feel satiated, which may allow you to cut calories by eating less during your meal. The probiotic compounds in acetic acid could be part of the reason some people feel the balsamic vinegar makes them feel full. Balsamic vinegar also contains strains of probiotic bacteria that enable healthy digestion and improve the health of the gut or microbiome. The gut microbiome is the collection of bacteria, protozoa and fungi, and their respective living systems in the gastrointestinal tract.[60] Your gut microbiome can be modified based on how you add to your diet. **Balsamic vinegar and extra-virgin olive oil should be key components to your diet to help with digestion.**

You can also use olive oil when you cook. The smoke point of olive oil is somewhere around 374–405 degrees, making it a safe choice for most cooking methods, including sautéing and pan frying.[61] [62]

If you need a healthy oil with a higher smoke point, you can use avocado oil which has a smoke point of 520 degrees *(App 4-1 Ref.)*. This may be necessary for high temperature vegetable stir-fry in a wok. Avocado oil is healthy and is a pale green oil rich in monounsaturated fats, which can lower heart disease and stroke risks. (Figure 8) Avocado oil has an anti-inflammatory effect, reducing CRP.[63] It's also a good source of the antioxidant vitamin E and has 70% monounsaturated fat. Avocado oil could be the healthiest cooking oil due to its low levels of polyunsaturated fat. Vegetable oils such as canola, soybean or corn oils are highly refined and considered inflammatory due to their high omega-6 content. Avocado oil also contains naturally occurring compounds called phytosterols. Phytosterols are structurally similar to cholesterol and can actually prevent some cholesterol from being absorbed. The drawback is that avocado oil has about 120 calories in a teaspoon. In comparison, olive oil has only 40 calories in a teaspoon. Therefore, you should consider the calories in avocado oil when using it. This is also the primary reason that you should use olive oil when cooking at a temperature lower than 400 degrees. Another problem with avocado oil is that many people are allergic to avocados, eliminating that as an option. These issues make extra-virgin olive oil the king of oils. It should be incorporated into your anti-inflammatory diet in as many ways as possible.

Another way to incorporate extra-virgin olive oil into your diet is to drink a teaspoon whenever you are hungry between meals. The oil will curb your appetite and hold you over to your next meal. It is only 40 calories per teaspoon and has fewer calories than most other snacks. Most individuals will prefer to take the extra-virgin olive oil with something else. You could soak the extra-virgin olive oil onto a small piece of multigrain or Ezekiel bread. A great option is to put some crushed garlic and salt in olive oil and use it as a dip with some petite carrots, broccoli or red pepper strips. You could make up a small shake with some green tea, fruit such as blueberries, and add some extra-virgin olive oil and place into a blender. Extra-virgin olive oil is great mixed with crushed garlic as a sandwich spread on multigrain bread or instead of pizza sauce on a homemade pizza.

Extra-virgin olive oil can also be added to your diet by adding it to soups, steel cut oatmeal, turkey chili, salmon spreads, and scrambled eggs. Try to add small amounts (one teaspoon) to many meals to enhance the anti-inflammatory benefits of the meals. Even if you purchase a soup, chili or other food from a restaurant you can add a teaspoon of extra-virgin olive oil to enhance the anti-inflammatory benefits.

Sesame oil, ghee and butter

Sesame oil also has some beneficial properties and can be incorporated into your diet. Sesame oil is rich in phytosterols and is known to block LDL cholesterol and help to reverse or prevent atherosclerosis.[64] Sesame oil has been shown to help decrease inflammation because of sesamol and sesaminol, two anti inflammatories. Sesame oil can also be used topically to decrease pain and improve healing. It contains 82% unsaturated fatty acids and is a healthy oil.

Sesame oil can form some unhealthy by-products if cooked at higher temperatures despite its relatively high smoke point. It also has relatively high omega-6 content, a poor characteristic. So your use of sesame oil should be limited to certain dishes. Edamame is great when cooked with sesame oil and sesame seeds *(App 4-2 AIF)*. To prepare, defrost the edamame and place in a frying pan with sesame oil after heating up on medium heat. Add some red pepper flakes and then add the edamame and heat until slightly browned. Add soy sauce and heat until most of the soy sauce has cooked into the edamame. Add some sesame seeds and serve hot. This is a very enjoyable snack that is healthy and anti-inflammatory.

Ghee is clarified butter, made by simmering the butter slowly to remove any milk solids and water. Ghee is more concentrated fat than butter but is free of milk sugar lactose and may be a better choice for those with lactose intolerance. Ghee has a higher smoke point of 485 degrees and can be used to pan fry at higher temperatures. However, ghee has a similar nutritional profile as butter with higher levels of saturated fats. If you have a higher LDL level you should avoid using butter or ghee in your diet.

	Ghee	Butter
Calories	112	100
Fat	13 grams	11 grams
Saturated fat	8 grams	7 grams
Monounsaturated fat	4 grams	3 grams
Polyunsaturated fat	0.5 grams	0.5 grams
Protein	Trace amounts	Trace amounts
Carbs	Trace amounts	Trace amounts
Vitamin A	12% of the Daily Value (DV)	11% of the DV
Vitamin E	2% of the DV	2% of the DV
Vitamin K	1% of the DV	1% of the DV

Taken from Healthline "Ghee: Is It Healthier than Regular Butter?" ***(App 4-4 Ref.)***

Bottom line: Extra-virgin olive oil is the best oil for an anti-inflammatory diet or keto diet and has proven to be an integral part of a healthy lifestyle as it is one of the primary components of the Mediterranean diet.

5

GREEN TEA AND SUPPLEMENTS

One of the best ways to promote an anti-inflammatory state and curb your comorbidities is to drink green tea and add some key supplements to your diet. **Green tea has been shown to have a significant effect on nasal symptomatology, joint and back pain, heart disease, diabetes, and it can potentially help prevent cancer *(App 5-1 Ref.)*.** It has an abundance of polyphenols, with the flavonoids being the most important. The most important flavonoids are the catechins, which make up 80 to 90% of them.[65] The amount of catechins that are available is dependent on many factors including how the tea leaves are harvested, how the leaves are processed and how the tea is prepared. Where the leaves are grown and seasonal differences can also affect catechin levels in the tea leaves. To help prevent loss of polyphenols the tea leaves are heated rapidly, using steam to inactivate polyphenol oxidase.

Benefits of green tea

The health benefits of green tea depend on the bioavailability of the catechins after consumption. These active ingredients can be measured in blood and urine after consumption.[66] Green tea has been shown to include anti-inflammatory, antimicrobial, anti-carcinogenic and antioxidant properties, as well as cardiovascular benefits. Cancers that were reduced include breast, colorectal, esophageal, gastric, lung, ovarian, pancreatic and prostate cancers.[67][68]

The anti-inflammatory benefits of green tea have been most extensively studied in patients with rheumatoid arthritis and osteoarthritis. The studies show that catechins in green tea downregulate the inflammatory factors in the body. This effect can be dramatic. Patients with rheumatoid arthritis can show a dramatic improvement in their symptoms by drinking three glasses of green tea a day *(App 5-2 Ref.)*. Patients with other autoimmune disorders such as lupus and Sjorgren's disease can be improved by drinking green tea as well.

From a practical point of view, you could start the day with a cup of green tea instead of your morning cup of coffee. You can also use green tea as the base for your shake if you choose to make a shake for one of your meals. If you do not want caffeine, you can use decaffeinated green tea *(App 5-3 Rec.)*. A cup of green tea is also great after lunch if you need a small pick-me-up. Green tea has 12mg to 20mg of caffeine per cup depending on how concentrated it is when prepared. Coffee, on the other hand, has 40 mg to 120mg depending on whether it is a dark or light roast and how concentrated it is. Decaffeinated coffee has about 8mg of caffeine in a cup.

If you choose to drink green tea, I would recommend putting the green tea leaves in hot water and allowing them to steep. You can then drink the tea with the tea leaves, consuming some, if not all, of them *(App 5-4 Ref.)*. You will benefit from consuming the tea leaves in addition to the green tea, getting more of the anti-inflammatory benefits. The only drawback is that you will also consume more caffeine. If this is OK with you, then you might as well get the extra antioxidant effects of the green tea. In order to do this you will have to use specific types of green tea. You can also incorporate green tea leaves into your food preparations such as with steel cut oatmeal, protein shakes, ground turkey burgers, salads, etc.

Matcha green tea

Another form of green tea where you are consuming the tea leaves is matcha green tea, which has about 80mg of caffeine. Matcha green tea is specially grown and ground up tea leaves. Matcha has more health benefits than regular green tea leaves that are steeped, since you are consuming the entire leaf. It has a much higher caffeine content that ranges from 65mg to 100mg of caffeine depending on the amount of powder used in the tea. Typically matcha will provide a long-lasting energy (four to five hours) effect compared to coffee and will give a higher peak and quicker resolution of the caffeine effect (within three hours) *(App 5-5 Ref.)*). (Figure 9)

The primary benefit to drinking matcha is the larger quantity of anti-inflammatory ingredients. (Figure 10) "Drinking brewed green tea is a bit like boiling spinach, throwing away the spinach and just drinking the water," says Louise Cheadle, co-author of The Book of Matcha. "You will get some of the nutrients, but you're throwing away the best bit *(App 5-6 Rec.)*."

With matcha, you're drinking whole tea leaves. The tea bushes are grown in the shade, which increases the chlorophyll in the leaves, making them greener and full of nutrients. The leaves are picked by hand and then the stems and veins are removed. The leaves are then finely ground into a powder. Cheadle emphasizes, "The finest matcha comes from Japan, where it has been grown for centuries and forms part of the traditional Japanese tea ceremony." Like other green teas, matcha is high in catechins, which are anti-inflammatory and cancer fighting. However, matcha is particularly high in a catechin called EGCG (epigallocatechin gallate), which has potent anti-cancer properties. These nutrients have also shown to prevent heart disease, type-2 diabetes and promote weight loss. Data published in 2015 showed that a cup of brewed green tea had 25mg to 86mg of EGCG, whereas matcha provided 17mg to 109mg of EGCG per serving *(App 5-7 Ref.)*. Matcha is more expensive and can range from $0.60 to $2.00 per serving depending on the quality. Higher-quality matcha will have a subtle sweetness and should be smooth like a good wine. There is a concern that since you are consuming the entire tea leaf there may be some harmful contaminants such as lead. However, studies have shown that most of the better brands of matcha have relatively low lead and PCB levels. **According to the USDA agricultural research service, gram for gram, matcha is one of the most powerful antioxidants** in nature. (Figure 11) So if you would like to decrease the inflammation in your body, have at least one cup of matcha green tea a day.

And a bonus: the matcha experience is second to none. If you ever have the opportunity to participate in a Japanese tea ceremony, you should do so. This was a very special event that focuses on the matcha tea preparation and the cherished drinking of the matcha. If you would like to benefit from the caffeine effects of the matcha, it is more potent than brewed green tea which typically has 12mg to 20mg of caffeine in a cup on average. A cup of matcha can have 40mg to 78mg of caffeine (50mg on average). Coffee can have 80mg to 135mg of caffeine (100mg on average) and will give you a rapid energy boost that may cause jitteriness and may end with an energy glut or "crash" after the caffeine effect wears off. Because the matcha leaf has the caffeine effect, it's prolonged as the matcha is digested. Matcha has unique forms of caffeine called theophylline and theobromine that are in the family of compounds called xanthines. Caffeine in matcha is more slowly absorbed in the presence of L-theanine and is released into the blood slowly. L-theanine is an important amino acid that enhances focus and mental stamina. It causes a significant increase in the α-waves (alpha waves) of the brain in the occipital and parietal regions, producing significant relaxation in the body, and reduces stress without any additional drowsiness or any form of impaired function. L-theanine also stimulates GABA and dopamine (the brain's naturally occurring "feel-good" chemical) to simultaneously increase focus and mood, while also reducing stress. Green tea (matcha is the highest) has a higher level of L-theanine over all other teas. Because of the L-theanine and its effect on alpha waves in the brain, it may also be a better choice than coffee for those who need to concentrate for long periods without the buzz. If you want a prolonged caffeine effect that lasts up to six hours, strongly consider the matcha option.

Other anti-Inflammatory teas

There are several other teas that are very healthy and anti-inflammatory *(App 5-8 Rec.)*. Teas with ginger and turmeric are very good and provide excellent anti-inflammatory benefits *(App 5-9*

Rec.). The active ingredient in turmeric is curcumin, which has been shown to decrease inflammation and has been effective in some skin cancer trials[69] The amount of curcumin gained is less than capsule supplements but still has benefits. Ginger teas have also been shown to have anti-inflammatory benefits as well as a gentle mild flavoring.[70] Ginger can also provide a calming effect to the gastrointestinal tract.

Black tea contains the polyphenol theaflavin, which has potent anti-inflammatory effects[71] Black tea comes in a wide variety, from classic black teas like English Breakfast, to the flavored black teas like Masala Chai and the Chinese black teas. When compared head to head, the green teas were found to have more of an anti-inflammatory effect due to the higher flavonoids (catechin) content.[72] Both green tea and black tea contain similar amounts of polyphenols, most notably the flavonoids. Their composition is different in green and black teas. Green tea contains more catechins (simple flavonoids), which promote the anti-inflammatory effects. However, black tea is still a very good anti-inflammatory supplement and may be taken in place of green tea. There are many different types of black tea produced in many areas of the world *(App 5-10 Ref.)*. Black tea is known as red tea in China and is very common.

White teas also have potent anti-inflammatory benefits.[73] White teas have lower caffeine levels and are a good option for those who would like to avoid the caffeine effects.

Chamomile teas have been shown to reduce inflammation as well.[74] Chamomile is a floral herbal tea that has been used as a remedy for muscle pain, colds, sleep issues and other illnesses. Chamomile can also help to give the immune system a boost and help improve overall health. Chamomile comes in many varieties of teas with different combinations of herbal additives that provide a great selection of flavorful choices. Chamomile teas should not be consumed if you are taking some antidepressants.

Rooibos tea is an herbal tea primarily grown in South Africa and is sometimes called red tea or red bush tea. Rooibos has a flavor similar to black tea and has a pleasant natural sweetness. This herbal tea is also caffeine-free, making it a great alternative for those that would like to avoid the effects of caffeine. Similar to black and green teas, rooibos also contains flavonoids, which have been shown to significantly reduce the symptoms of inflammation and oxidative stress.

As you can see, there are many options for teas that provide anti-inflammatory benefits. Some are with caffeine and some without. You should think about drinking teas throughout the day. You could replace your daily cup of coffee with a cup of tea instead. The teas without caffeine will not have a diuretic effect and can be taken during the day to help rehydrate your body. Even if you are unable to drink green tea or if you just do not like the taste of green tea, you can have one of these other options to provide the anti-inflammatory benefits from tea leaves. Most of you will be able to have the caffeine-containing tea (green and black) in the first half of the day and the no-caffeine options during the latter half of the day. If you do not add tea products to your diet, you are missing one of the most efficient means to decrease your body's inflammation, improve your general health, minimize your comorbidities and decrease the likelihood of having a more complicated course if you should contract Covid-19.

Supplements

Free radicals are constantly being formed in our bodies, and they attack molecules in our cells, potentially removing an electron. This creates an unstable molecule in the cell *(App 5-11 Ref. Video +)*. The unstable molecule is a free radical that can damage our cells by oxidizing lipids, proteins and DNA. Free radicals have an unpaired electron that destabilizes the molecule, allowing it to damage our cells. Free radicals form all of the time and are created from breathing, eating, exercising, etc. Specific things that cause free radicals to form include; stress, UV radiation, toxins and inflammatory foods. Free radicals can induce mutations in our cells, causing many disorders such as cancer, heart disease, Alzheimer's and autoimmune or inflammatory disorders (arthritis, lupus, psoriasis, etc.). Free radicals can steal an electron from other molecules in our cells forming another free radical. This chain reaction continues, resulting in oxidative stress in our bodies.

How can we stop the free radicals from damaging our cells and creating a damaging oxidative state? The answer is antioxidants, which can safely donate an electron to free radicals acting to neutralize the free radical before it can damage our cells. (Figure 12) It donates an electron to pair up with the unpaired electron, making it whole again. This halts the chain reaction that the free radicals can cause, stopping the further increase of free radicals in our cells. This stops the formation of degenerative diseases and slows the aging process. We must provide our bodies with essential antioxidants such as vitamin A, vitamin C, vitamin E, glutathione, beta-carotene and selenium. If the free radicals overwhelm the antioxidant capacity of our bodies, oxidative stress will occur.

If you primarily eat inflammatory foods you are taking electrons from molecules in your cells and propagating the formation of free radicals. If you overwhelm your body's anti-inflammatory defenses, your cells will be damaged by the free radicals, potentially causing diseases such as cancer, Alzheimer's, diabetes and heart disease. In essence, you create your own health problems.

Turmeric
Supplements such as turmeric can help with your anti-inflammatory diet. Turmeric is a spice that is used in many Indian foods and gives it the yellow color. Curcumin is the main active ingredient in turmeric and has very strong anti-inflammatory and anti-oxidative effects. The mechanism for curcumin's

anti-inflammatory and antioxidative effects is multifactorial.[75] Curcumin can scavenge multiple forms of free radicals by modulating multiple different enzymes. Curcumin is also thought to inhibit cyclooxygenase-2 (COX-2), lipoxygenase (LOX), and inducible nitric oxide synthase (iNOS), which are enzymes that mediate inflammatory processes. Increased activity of COX-2 and/or iNOS has been associated with certain types of human cancer as well as inflammatory disorders.[76]

Incorporating turmeric spice into your diet is a good way to gain some of the anti-inflammatory and antioxidant effects of curcumin. The actual amount of curcumin in the turmeric spice can vary tremendously. Pure turmeric powder has the highest levels of curcumin, which is only 3.14% by weight.[77] The most efficient way to add curcumin to your diet is to take curcumin supplements. Curcumin by itself has poor availability in the body primarily due to rapid metabolism in the intestinal wall and liver. If consumed with black pepper, the absorption is significantly increased. The active ingredient in the black pepper is piperine, which increases the absorption of the curcumin by 2000%.[78] The piperine inhibits the metabolism of the curcumin by the intestines and liver by slowing glucuronidation. This combination of curcumin and piperine dramatically enhances the availability of curcumin to the body. There are many curcumin supplements that are available on the market. You should choose one that has the piperine added to get the enhanced availability.

Choosing the right curcumin supplement to take can be very confusing. You should look for a curcumin formula containing at least 400mg of curcumin infused with standardized 95% curcuminoid. Curcumin is fat soluble and is poorly absorbed, limiting bioavailability unless taken with fat or pepper. If the formula has Bioperine, absorption can be increased by 2000% *(App 5-12 Ref.)*. Some formulas do not have Bioperine but contain another compound to increase absorption. Also avoid formulas that contain yellow dye such as Acid Yellow 36. You should also take a formula that has been tested for lead levels as many types of turmeric from India can be contaminated with lead, which is a known neurotoxin that can damage the brain, heart and kidneys. Recommendations on which brand or formula to choose will likely change with time and therefore, no singular recommendation can be made *(App 5-13 Rec. +)*. Another means of getting curcumin is to consume one tablespoon of the turmeric spice a day *(App 5-14 Ref. Video +)*. This will have about 1000mg of curcumin and should be taken with black pepper to increase absorption.

Omega-3 supplements

There are many other supplements that can decrease inflammation in your body. Omega-3 supplements are also anti-inflammatory and are broken down into two major categories. There are the long chain omega-3 fatty acids that contain eicosapentaenoic acid (EPA) and docosahexaenoic acid (DHA), precursors of certain eicosanoids that are plentiful in fish, shellfish and some forms of algae. The other major form is the shorter chain omega-3 fatty acids such as alpha-linolenic acid (ALA), which are found in plants such as flax seed. The EPA and DHA have much more anti-inflammatory properties than ALA. As previously mentioned, omega-3 fatty acids are anti-inflammatory whereas the omega-6 fatty acids are inflammatory. Unfortunately, the average diet in the United States has 20 times more omega-6 fatty acids compared to omega-3 fatty acids. This is one of the reasons there is so much chronic disease and why so many people are constantly in an inflamed state. It's also one of the reasons that many people have multiple comorbidities. DHA is one of the most prevalent fatty acids in the brain. **In a study of 800 men and women ages 65 to 94, those who ate fish at least once a week were much less likely to develop Alzheimer's disease.**[79]

In addition to eating wild caught salmon you can take omega-3 fish oil capsules. Omega-3 inhibits cyclooxygenase, which triggers inflammation. Omega-3 fatty acids also decrease the production of inflammatory eicosanoids, cytokines, and reactive oxygen species and the expression of adhesion molecules.[80] You can take omega-3 fish oil capsules daily to decrease your body's inflammation. You should choose a supplement that is relatively pure and is clear of PCBs and mercury. Omega-3 and omega-6 fatty acids compete for the same binding site on the COX-1 enzyme that converts the omega-6 fatty acids to prostaglandin. Prostaglandins are naturally occurring hormone-like substances that can accentuate inflammation and thrombosis. The more omega-3 fatty acids that are available to block the COX-1 enzyme binding sites, the fewer omega-6 fatty acids are able to be converted to prostaglandin. Even though some of the omega-3 acids can be converted to prostaglandins, those formed from omega-3 are much less potent and therefore less harmful.[81] Omega-3 fatty acids in fish oil have also been found to reduce the risk of heart disease and decrease blood pressure and triglycerides while increasing high-density lipoproteins (HDL), improving autoimmune disorders and relieving symptoms of rheumatoid arthritis *(App 5-14 Ref. Video +)*.

Taking fish oil can cause some side effects such as upset stomach, nausea, rash and increased chance of bleeding. The fish oil supplements can interact with blood thinning agents such as anticoagulants and antiplatelet drugs accentuating the potential for bleeding. Check with your physician before starting to take fish oil supplements. When you take fish oil you also may note the fishy aftertaste. Many of these issues can be avoided if you choose the right fish oil supplement. Some guidelines recommend taking from 250mg to 500mg of combined EPA and DHA each day for healthy adults *(App 5-16 Ref.)*. These doses can be increased significantly for people with certain disorders. For example, patients with heart disease take 1,000mg of combined EPA and DHA daily, while those with high triglycerides take 2,000–4,000mg daily.[82] The Food and Drug Administration (FDA) states that omega-3 supplements containing EPA and DHA are safe if doses don't exceed 3,000mg per day.

There are several options for fish oil on the market. You can get natural fish oil or processed fish oil. The amount of omega-3 fatty acid in natural fish oils varies from 18% to 31%.[83] Natural fish oils also provide vitamin A and vitamin E. Most fish oil on the market is processed and is purified or concentrated. The process of purification eliminates impurities such as mercury and PCBs. This is important as these contaminants can be very harmful. Mercury is particularly harmful to the fetus and should be avoided in pregnant mothers. Many of the processed fish oils have concentrated the EPA and DHA to levels up to 50 to 90%. Processed fish oils can come in ethyl ester or triglyceride forms (triglycerols). The ethyl ester forms are less easily absorbed, are less stable and can oxidize more rapidly, becoming rancid. The triglyceride forms of processed fish oil are more stable and more easily absorbed.[84] These are also referred to as reesterified triglycerides. They are highly resorbed, but are also more expensive.

Selecting an omega-3 fatty acid supplement is very difficult as there are so many options on the market. You can purchase omega-3 supplements online, at your local grocer, or at health food stores. Many of these companies make several claims that are unsubstantiated. When choosing an omega-3 fatty acid supplement you should choose one that has been purified so mercury and PCBs are removed. It should have the recommended daily dose of 1500mg omega-3 fish oil, which includes 800mg EPA and 600mg DHA. Ideally, the preparation should come from cold-water oily fish, such as salmon, mackerel, anchovies and sardines. Oils from these fish have around seven times as many omega-3 fatty acids than other fish. If the company uses a third party to test its product, that would be the most reliable means to ensure safety and efficacy. There are some omega-3 supplements on the market that fit these parameters and would be good choices *(App 5-17 Rec.)*. If cost is important to you, there are some lower-priced options that are acceptable. These will tend to have lower concentrations of EPA and DHA but are still good for you. I believe some of the more reliable omega-3 fatty acid supplements have been around for a while and have developed a strong reputation while maintaining good supply *(App 5-18 Rec. +)*. Some of the vendors have variable stock and are frequently out of product. At minimum, you should make sure the omega-3 supplement that you choose has filtered out mercury and PCBs and has a minimum of 500mg of EPA and DHA.

Krill oil is marketed as another source for omega-3 fatty acids. Even though krill oils have a phospholipid omega-3 based oil, which makes it much easier to absorb into your body, the levels of DHA and EPA are relatively low. A high quality omega-3 fish oil supplement will contain approximately 500% more DHA and EPA compared to krill oil. Krill oil also includes astaxanthin, a potent antioxidant not found in fish oils.[85] However, the levels of astaxanthin are relatively low as well. This would require you to take a very large amount of krill oil to gain the benefits of concentrated omega-3 fish oil capsules.

Resveratrol

Resveratrol is an antioxidant found in blueberries, grapes, red wine and peanuts that has been shown to have potent anti-inflammatory properties. It also helps patients with cardiovascular disease, arthritis, ulcerative colitis and diabetes.[86][87] There is resveratrol in red wine, but in relatively small amounts. There are approximately 1.5mg to 13mg per liter of red wine. To gain the beneficial effect of resveratrol you will need to consume 150mg per day or more than 11 liters of wine per day. To reach the higher concentration of resveratrol you would have to drink 750 to 1,500 bottles of red wine per day. This is obviously not possible, so you can take resveratrol capsules. However, there is not a lot of research on the benefits of resveratrol capsules taken in higher doses. Therefore, it may be better to just eat a lot of blueberries and have an occasional glass of red wine.

Pomegranate juice

Pomegranate juice is a potent anti-inflammatory agent that is loaded with antioxidant polyphenols that can help to decrease inflammation, remove free radicals and protect from cell damage.[88] The anti-aging effects of pomegranate are notable in helping to repair damaged skin. Pomegranate juice has even more antioxidants than green tea and is loaded with vitamin C, vitamin E, vitamin K and folate. A half cup of pomegranate juice contains 16 grams of sugar and 75 calories. This is a moderate amount of sugar, but as long as the juice you buy has no added sugar it will be the natural sugar of the fruit. Despite the sugar, pomegranate juice has been shown to help those with arthritis by decreasing their joint pain.[89] Pomegranate juice has also been shown to be beneficial in fighting prostate cancer.[90]

Pomegranate juice helps to control hypertension by reducing levels of Angiotensin-converting enzyme (ACE), which is an important protein that helps to control the size of blood vessels.[91] You can add a shot of pomegranate juice to your shake to increase the antioxidant value of your breakfast drink. You can also enjoy eating the pomegranate fruit itself. It can be a chore, but it is flavorful *(App 5-19 AIF Video +)*. You should break up the pomegranate in a bowl of water to gently separate the seeds from the rest of the fruit. You can eat the seeds with no problems; however, most of us prefer to discard the seeds. If you eat the seeds, you will gain a tremendous amount of fiber. The pomegranate seeds are called "arils." You can get a pomegranate deseeder, which will remove the seeds so you can enjoy them with no fibrous shell. Great ways to incorporate pomegranate seeds into your diet is to put them on your salads, add them to a cool summer drink, put them in a shake or just eat them as snacks. You can refrigerate them for a day or two or even freeze them and defrost when you are ready to eat.

There are many other anti-inflammatory supplements that are available on the market. However, I would limit to incorporating green tea, curcumin and omega-3 fish oil as the primary supplements to decrease the inflammation in your body.

6

THE IMPACT OF EXERCISE ON YOUR IMMUNE SYSTEM AND COVID-19 OUTCOME

Exercise has many beneficial effects on your body in addition to the positive effects on your immune system and cardiovascular system.[92] Chronic low-grade inflammation is a common manifestation of aging and is associated with a significant increase in pro-inflammatory cytokines such as interleukin 6 (IL-6), tumor necrosis factor (TNF) and C-reactive protein (CRP).[93] During exercise, your muscle cells release IL-6, which is also thought to play an important role in fighting inflammation.[94] IL-6 has several anti-inflammatory effects, including decreasing levels of TNF-alpha (tumor necrosis factor-alpha) which triggers inflammation in the body.[95] It is evident that IL-6 has pro-inflammatory and anti-inflammatory properties.[96]

The amount of IL-6 that is released into your body depends on the length and level of intensity of your workout. If you work out for 30 minutes your IL-6 levels will increase five-fold. A more intense workout using larger muscle mass will increase the IL-6 levels to a greater extent.[97] The amount of IL-6 that is produced in your body will increase significantly if you work out for over an hour using the larger muscles in your legs (running or climbing stairs).

During exercise the brain and nervous system are activated to release epinephrine and norepinephrine. These compounds trigger receptors in immune cells and block the TNF-alpha. Researchers found that a single 20-minute session on a treadmill resulted in a 5% reduction in the stimulated cells producing TNF-alpha *(App 6-1 Ref.)*.[98] This 20-minute session on the treadmill was adjusted based on the study participant's fitness level. This study showed that you do not need to exercise intensely to gain the anti-inflammatory benefits. This is an important piece of information for those who may be intimidated by the thought of maximal high-intensity workout sessions.

Studies have also shown that exercise increases levels of extracellular superoxide dismutase (EcSOD), which helps to protect against acute respiratory distress syndrome (ARDS).[99] ARDS is a condition where the inflammation in the lungs becomes severe and the lung tissues become stiff, swollen and leaky, with fluid buildup to the point where oxygenation becomes difficult. This is why many Covid-19 patients who are in an intensive care unit need to be placed on a ventilator to help them breathe. The Centers for Disease Control reports that 20% to 42% of patients hospitalized with Covid-19 will develop ARDS. EcSOD can neutralize free radicals that cause inflammation in the lungs and other organs. Regular exercise can build up levels of EcSOD that can help to prevent the inflammation in the lungs seen in severe cases of Covid-19 *(App 6-2 Ref.)*. A combination of aerobic and weight training appears to provide the most significant increases in EcSOD. The research shows that even a single session of exercise will increase EcSOD levels. However, to gain significant increases in EcSOD, regular exercise is necessary.

Review of a number of clinical studies on the benefits of regular exercise and inflammation has revealed that exercise results in a decrease in systemic markers of inflammation.[100] These studies clearly demonstrate the anti-inflammatory benefits of exercise. This benefit is particularly important in the older individuals who are predisposed to higher levels of inflammation with inactivity.

Over-exercising can create increased inflammation and in the absence of periods of rest you may become locally inflamed *(App 6-3 Ref.)*. If your muscles are overworked, you may start to damage muscles and, if not given a period of time to heal and recover, the inflammation in the muscles can persist. Intense exercise during an infection can have a detrimental effect on the progression of the infection.[101] In the Gene Smart Anti-inflammatory Diet and Exercise Program, diet is combined with exercise in an effort to decrease whole body inflammation *(App 6-4 Ref.)*. The Gene Smart program recommends working out four to five times a week for at least 30 minutes. The week is broken down into two days of weight training and three days of aerobic exercise (walking, running or swimming). With the aerobic exercise, the goal is to get your heart rate to 70% to 85% of maximum. The weight training is designed to work 8 to 10 muscle groups.

Another major benefit of exercise is its effect on mood. Exercise can help depression by increasing serotonin levels that help your body regulate mood, sleep and appetite. Exercise also increases endorphins which act to elevate your mood. A burst of endorphins makes many people feel euphoric. Exercise will decrease cortisol, which is a stress hormone that can injure your body and damage your brain cells (hippocampus). It is clear that exercise can help patients with depression and may be more effective than many antidepressant medications *(App 6-5 Ref.)*. Exercise will tend to elevate your mood and actually make you more likely to adhere to an anti-inflammatory diet because you will feel better and have more positive thoughts. You may become dependent on the "euphoric" feelings you get with exercise and work out more often to achieve that state.

If you do not exercise you're more likely to feel depressed, and your energy level will drop, which will make it harder to adhere to the diet. A vicious cycle of chronic inflammation can be set in motion as the inactivity increases abdominal fat, which in turn promotes development of depression and poor mood. The inactivity promotes muscle loss and tiredness, which in turn leads to more inactivity and no drive to move. This inactivity will result in further deconditioning and increases in stress hormones.

The atrophy of the muscles and increased inflammation affect cardiovascular performance and the ability to exercise.[102] Physical inactivity can also result in heart disease, a major comorbidity that increases the risk of a poor outcome if one acquires Covid-19. Infection by SARS-CoV-2 can result in damage to the heart muscle and permanent scarring.[103] A healthy heart muscle is better able to manage the stresses of the viral infection.

Closing of fitness centers and parks resulted in decreased physical activity. This decrease in physical activity can weaken the immune system and its antiviral defenses.[104] Experiments in animals exposed to viral infections showed that moderate exercise before and during the infection improved morbidity and mortality to the infection.[105] Physical activity and exercise have been shown to increase efficiency of leukocytes (infection fighting cells) and likely increases the body's ability to fight off viruses after exposure.[106]

Once one is infected with SARS-CoV-2 and needs to go on a ventilator, those who have exercised regularly have a diaphragm (muscle that moves the lungs) that is preconditioned to do better if placed on a ventilator.[107] It is predicted that endurance trained individuals that develop Covid-19 and are placed on a ventilator will benefit from the exercise-related preconditioning of the diaphragm muscle *(App 6-6 Ref.)*.

Skeletal muscle inactivity can result in an increase in insulin resistance and increased inflammation.[108] This shift in use of glucose and insulin will increase abdominal visceral fat stores. Significant muscle atrophy has been noted in 14 days of inactivity. This muscle inactivity can result in a decline in mitochondrial function. The mitochondria are the powerhouse of energy stores. This can result in increases in systemic inflammation and lead to less ideal Covid-19 outcomes *(App 6-7 Ref.)*.

Can physical fitness help you prevent infection by SARS-CoV-2 or improve your likelihood of a good outcome after getting infected? There is presently no data that shows that the level of physical fitness affects the progress of Covid-19. However, it is well documented that a strong immune system could affect the severity of the Covid-19 infection.[109] Depression related to prolonged isolation or inactivity can result in a weakening of the immune system, which in turn can make you more vulnerable to the SARS-CoV-2 virus. Exercise has powerful antidepressive effects and is related to brain derived neurotrophic factor (BDNF). The negative effects of depression on the brain can be noted in the hippocampus, which is important to memory, stress regulation and emotional processing. As noted earlier, exercise can increase endorphins, creating a euphoric feeling and help to combat quarantine-induced depression or Covid-19 related emotional trauma. Moderate to intense exercise has been shown to increase endorphin levels, whereas low-intensity exercise does not create this effect.[110] This overarching effect of exercise may be one of the most important factors in the prevention of severe disease when contracting Covid-r19.

Types of exercise

There are many types of exercise that you can incorporate into your weekly routine to decrease your bodies inflammation. Taking 20-minute or longer walks can decrease your inflammation *(App 6-8 Ref.)*. You can count steps using a digital pedometer or equivalent device.

*Steps	2 mph (slow) 60 steps/min	5 mph (fast) 100 steps/min
2,000	33	20
3,000	50	30
4,000	67	40
5,000	83	50

(App 6-9 Ref.)

Walking after a meal is a great way to improve digestion, work off some calories and decrease inflammation. Walking is low impact and can be easily incorporated into your day. You can take the stairs instead of the elevator. Swimming is an excellent low-impact aerobic exercise that will work many of your larger muscles and is great for cardiovascular health. Sports such as tennis and soccer are excellent aerobic exercises. If you play golf, be sure to walk as much as possible to get some aerobic benefit.

Resistance training is another excellent means to work your muscles *(App 6-10 Rec.)*. There are many programs that are available that incorporate simple equipment such as resistance bands and light weights *(App 6-11 Rec.)*. There are also intense workouts if you are very fit *(App 6-12 Rec. Video)*.

Simply doing push-ups, sit-ups and pull-ups can significantly increase your muscle strength *(App 6-13 Rec.)*. There are also pull-up bar programs that are excellent for increasing your core strength and toning your abdominal muscles *(App 6-14 Rec. Video +)*.

There are a series of relatively easy core exercises that you can do several times a week that can do wonders for your core and also to decrease abdominal fat *(App 6-15 Rec. +)*. Simply doing sit-ups will likely not do the trick. Crunches work out a limited number of the muscles of your core. It is important to work the muscles of your lower back, hips, and upper thighs.

Boring core muscle exercises such as the plank help train more of your core muscles to stabilize the spine and pelvis. This will also help to improve your back and spine regions and possibly improve your back problems. Plank-type exercises also burn more calories because they work more muscles of your core. A good series of plank exercises that are easy to perform are noted in the *New Rules of Lifting for Abs* *(App 6-16 Rec. +)*. In their book, Schuler and Cosgrove explain how typical crunches only work on the rectus abdominis muscles and some of the obliques but do not work your entire core *(App 6-17 Rec. +)*.[111] By implementing a series of more difficult plank-type exercises, you will be able to strengthen your entire core and better support your back and spine. A few of the best and simplest plank-like exercises include the following.

The side plank is very simple and involves supporting your body weight at two contact points, requiring your core muscles to support your body. To properly execute this maneuver, you lie on your side and place your elbow under your shoulder on the floor; your legs should be side by side. Place your opposite hand on your opposite hip. You should try to hold this position for 30 to 60 seconds and then switch to the opposite side and repeat several times. The next plank maneuver involves the Paloff press with your opposite hand straight in the air and with your legs spread. You should hold this position for the same 30 to 60 seconds and repeat on the other side.

The next step is the walk-out to push-up. In this maneuver you will get into a push-up position. Then gradually walk your hands outward as far as possible then walk them back to just under your shoulders. You can also walk your legs outward as you walk your arms out to add a bit more difficulty. You should do 10 to 13 reps each time. The fourth maneuver is the alligator drag, where you start in a push-up position with your toes set on a sliding object such as a plastic disk. If you have two tops of a jar or two small plates, that works great if they will slide easily over a carpeted floor. With your tips of your feet on the jar tops you should walk with your hands and arms across the floor for 10 to 20 yards and then walk backwards to where you started. These four plank exercises are simple yet effective in working your core muscles. This will burn more calories and better tone your midsection. It will transform your core workout and provide a more comprehensive program to decrease your abdominal girth. You do not need a lot of fancy equipment to maximally work out your abdomen and core muscles. However, there are some exercise devices that can help engage you and push you through your core workout *(App 6-18 Rec. +)*. If you need some help getting motivated, some of these methods may help.

Yoga has been found to be helpful in decreasing your waistline.[112] Some of the most beneficial yoga maneuvers include the warrior

III roll-ups, down dog hip rolls, forearm plank hip taps, boat low repetitions, half moon, revolved half moon, side angle reverse warrior flows and high lunge twists. In addition to strengthening your core muscles, yoga will help to reduce your stress and decrease cortisol in your body *(App 6-20 Ref.)*.[113] Cortisol acts to increase fat around your midsection.[114] By reducing cortisol levels you can more readily decrease the size of your waistline.

Pilates is also an excellent form of exercise to decrease inflammation by improving lymphatic flow and strengthening muscles *(App 6-21 Ref.)*. Pilates promotes proper breathing and core work, along with supported movement to help lubricate joint surfaces, providing nutrition to the cartilage *(App 6-22 Ref.)*. Smooth, pain-free body movement can help reduce total body inflammation.

Tai Chi can decrease stress and lower cortisol levels.[115] Meditation has also been shown to help with decreasing stress in your life. Virtually any ritual or activity that lowers your stress levels will help you in the process of reducing your waistline.

Older individuals are at the highest risk for a suboptimal outcome after contracting Covid-19, and this group will benefit the most from increasing their physical activity and exercise. Moderate intensity aerobic exercise for two to three sessions a week not less than 30 minutes is the minimum to gain beneficial brain effects.

Bottom line: Exercise helps to minimize inflammation. Even more important is to avoid increases in abdominal fat as the health effects are very detrimental, increasing your likelihood of becoming diabetic and/or developing heart disease or contracting a chronic disease such as Alzheimer's disease.[116] Minimizing or eliminating comorbidities could be key to surviving the next Covid-9 pandemic. Incorporate exercise to elevate your mood and help you achieve a healthier state: the anti-inflammatory state.

7
YOUR WAISTLINE TELLS THE STORY

Many of us tend to gain weight around our mid-section during the holidays or when we are stressed. During the pandemic, many of us were stressed, ate a lot of comfort foods, and did not exercise. The result was increased abdominal girth. This is a result of increases in subcutaneous fat and/or visceral fat. (Figure 13) Visceral fat is a bigger problem and is a more important indicator of general health *(App 7-1 Ref.)*. Increased visceral fat is associated with your stress response mechanisms and can release harmful products that can increase blood pressure, raise blood sugar levels and increase your risk of heart disease.[117] Unlike subcutaneous fat, which has no particularly bad effects other than making your clothes fit too tightly, visceral fat cells are enlarged with excess triglycerides and release harmful metabolic products that flow to the liver, pancreas, heart and other organs. This can result in organ dysfunction and resultant heart disease and diabetes. These co-morbidities are linked to a poor outcome if you should contract Covid-19.

However, some research indicates that a slimmer waistline is associated with a longer lifespan.[118] **In a study of 48,500 men and 56,343 women over age 50, having a large waist size doubled the risk of dying.** A large waist circumference was associated with higher risk of mortality among both men and women. Independent of BMI being normal, overweight or obese, avoiding gains in waist circumference reduced the risk of early mortality *(App 7-2 Ref.)*. In the study, "associations with waist circumference were strongest for mortality caused by respiratory disease, followed by cardiovascular disease and then cancer." Coincidentally, these comorbidities are also associated with higher morbidity rates for those who contract Covid-19.

Measuring visceral fat

Determining how much visceral fat you have is difficult because it lies inside of your abdomen. It can be easily measured with a radiologic scan of the abdomen, but this is not likely to be ordered by your doctor. There are several ways to measure your abdominal fat that you can do yourself. You can measure your waist-to-hip ratio. You can measure your waistline at the level of the navel with your abdomen relaxed (not pulling your stomach in). Then measure your hips at the widest point, near the bony prominences of your hip bone. Then divide the waist size by your hip size to get the ratio of waist to hip size (waist in inches/hips in inches). Your risk of suffering a stroke or heart attack is increased if this ratio rises above 0.95 in a male or 0.85 in a female *(App 7-3 Ref.)*.

A simpler method is to simply measure your waist circumference using a tape measure. In a relaxed state, gently exhale and measure your waist at the level of your navel. Make sure you are not holding your stomach in or inhaling. For a male, you are at low risk if you measure out at 37 inches or less, intermediate risk at 37.1 inches to 39.9 inches, and high risk at 40 inches or above *(App 7-4 Ref.)*. For a woman, you are low risk at 31.5 inches or less, intermediate risk from 31.6 inches to 34.9 inches, and high risk at 35 inches or above.

Despite using these measurements, you may still have visceral fat that you are not aware of. In fact, you may have a relatively flat tummy area yet have a lot of visceral fat surrounding your abdominal organs. The only way to know for sure is to get an MRI or CT scan of your abdomen to evaluate the amount of fat surrounding your organs. Losing weight will tend to decrease visceral fat. However, if you are already in a proper weight range and cannot afford to lose weight, then your only option is to eat healthier. That means cutting saturated fats and going onto the anti-inflammatory diet. If you are able to decrease your visceral fat you will likely decrease your comorbidities, improve your likelihood of doing well if you should contract Covid-19 and lessen your chance of dying from heart disease or stroke.

Hormones and fat

As we age, we will have a tendency to increase subcutaneous abdominal fat and increase the size of our waistline. This is in part due to a decrease in estrogen in women and a decrease in testosterone in men. These hormones begin to decrease when you reach your 40s. An option is to take replacement hormones to elevate these depleted hormone levels. Signs of low testosterone in men include depression, disturbed sleep, increased body fat, declining muscle mass, lower sex drive and general fatigue. Women may experience depression, painful sex, or irregular periods. There are distinct risks of taking hormone replacement. If you take testosterone, you may have increased risk of heart attack, stroke or prostate cancer.[119] Other annoying but non-life-threatening symptoms include acne, disturbed sleep and breast swelling. Risks for women taking estrogen include increased risk of blood clots and stroke, endometrial cancer and potential dementia. Annoying but non-life-threatening symptoms include breast tenderness, fluid retention and irregular vaginal bleeding. Another big problem with taking testosterone replacement is that once you start taking testosterone, your body will stop making it and you may get stuck on testosterone replacement *(App 7-5 Ref.+)*. Our focus in this chapter is to show you how to decrease your abdominal fat without resorting to hormone replacement.

Thankfully, there are natural ways to increase your hormone levels without resorting to taking hormone replacement. In men and women, testosterone can be increased by lifting weights regularly.[120] High-intensity interval training was also shown to increase testosterone levels *(App 7-6 Ref. +)*.[121]

As cortisol levels increase with elevated stress, testosterone levels can decrease. Cortisol has been shown to block testosterone's effects *(App 7-7 Ref.)*. High cortisol levels can result in loss of fertility, decreased libido and increased abdominal fat. High cortisol levels can create a clinical picture of low testosterone despite having normal testosterone blood levels. Easier said than done, but by lowering your stress you can help to prevent lowering of your testosterone levels. Testosterone-lowering foods include processed foods, mint, vegetable oils (canola oil), soy-based products, flax seed and alcohol *(App 7-8 Ref.)*. Testosterone levels can be increased by increasing your vitamin D levels.[122] **Nearly half of us in the United States are deficient in vitamin D**.[123] In a 12-month study of 200 subjects, testosterone levels were increased by approximately 25% by taking 3,000 units of vitamin D per day. Zinc has also been shown to increase testosterone levels.[124] Foods high in zinc include oysters, red meats and vegetables such as mushrooms and kale. Legumes such as chickpeas and lentils are a good source of zinc. You can add edamame as well as it is high in zinc. Nuts such as pine nuts and pumpkin seeds are relatively high in zinc.

Getting good sleep is also important to keeping your testosterone levels higher. Some other natural means of increasing your testosterone levels include taking D-aspartic acid, ginger and dehydroepiandrosterone (DHEA) *(App 7-9 Ref. +)*. You can try to add ginger to your diet and take 3,000 units of vitamin D per day. Ashwagandha is an herb that acts to fight inflammation and lower blood sugar *(App 7-10 Rec.)*. It also helps you manage stress by decreasing cortisol.[125] Ashwagandha has a potent effect on increasing testosterone levels.[126] Other herbs or compounds that can boost testosterone include horny goat weed (epimedium grandiflorum), tribulus terrestris, mucuna pruriens, panax quinquefolius, cordyceps mushroom, euryooma, longifolla shilajit and tongkat ali. There are many supplements that contain different combinations of these ingredients *(App 7-11 Rec.)*. Consult your physician before taking these supplements.

Diet and exercise: keys to cutting subcutaneous fat

For those of us who would like to decrease our subcutaneous fat, we have several options. First and foremost is to try to cut back on calories. If you can cut your caloric intake by 25% you will set yourself on the correct path to losing abdominal fat (subcutaneous and visceral). If you need a number, you should try to cut about 500 calories to 750 calories a day to lose 1 pound to 1 1/2 pounds a week. Most dietitians agree that it takes approximately a 3,500-calorie reduction to burn off one pound of stored fat in your body. This drop in calories and body weight will help to shrink fat cells and decrease the size of the fat component of your abdomen. You would benefit from creating a meal plan that contains 40% complex carbohydrates, 30% protein and 30% good fats (monounsaturated fats). These numbers will be different if you choose to go on the anti-inflammatory diet with the keto push. That means you will be eating a lot of vegetables such as broccoli, cauliflower, asparagus, green beans and artichokes. You can also have a nice size salad with lunch and dinner. This will help to fill you up and make you satiated earlier. The proteins should be low in saturated fats and preferably anti-inflammatory. Chicken, fish, lean meats, beans and tofu are great options. Keep the skin off of the chicken and eat primarily organic free-range chicken and grass-fed beef. Eat wild, not farm-raised, fish.

Many weight loss programs tout protein shakes as a means of losing weight by replacing a meal with a shake. Starting the day with a protein shake has been shown to decrease caloric intake later in the day.[127] The green tea and blueberry shake with ground flax seed, chia seeds and egg white protein is a good option for many reasons. In a study it was shown that drinking three cups of green tea a day provided a reduction in weight, lower BMI and a reduced waist circumference.[128]

One of the quickest ways to improve your mid-section is to stop alcohol intake. Many of you may have a glass of wine or a couple of beers with dinner. You might think that a glass of red wine has health benefits, but when you look at it critically, the benefits of the red wine are miniscule and are likely outweighed by the calories and problems it can create with sleep and dehydration.

In order to gain the benefits of resveratrol in the red wine, you would have to drink several bottles a day. When people drink, they are adding empty calories that have little benefit. So you are really left with the sugar and calories that can go directly to your waistline. Additionally, when you drink alcohol you tend to make poor choices such as eating fatty inflammatory foods. So the first step is to stop or at least cut back on the alcohol. By cutting the alcohol you could cut hundreds, maybe thousands, of calories. You will also sleep better, feel better, be better hydrated and decrease your propensity for diabetes and liver disease. The potential effect on your immune system is also significant, which will improve your ability to fight off SARS-CoV-2.

On the fitness side, strength training is very important, and there are specific exercises you can do to help improve your waistline. These were discussed in detail in Chapter 6.

Spending time with family and friends can also help to lower stress levels.[129] Spending time with family and friends decreases stress by allowing you to leave stresses from work at the door and not bringing them into your home. Time with family and friends also helps to share tasks, as having meals together gives you a means of open communication. "Blue zone" is a non-scientific term given to geographic regions where a large number of people live to be over 100 years of age. Blue zones were initially described by Dan Buettner who studied these areas of the world and looked at what they had in common.[130] The blue zones include Icaria (Greece), Ogliastra, Sardinia (Italy), Okinawa (Japan), Nicoya Peninsula (Costa Rica) and Seventh-day Adventists in Loma Linda, California (USA). One of the common characteristics amongst the "Blue Zones" was staying connected to family and friends to decrease stress *(App 7-11 Rec.)*. Genetics was shown to contribute only about 20% to 30% of the role in longevity. Therefore, diet, lifestyle and environmental factors play a huge role in determining your lifespan. Connecting with family and friends is a big part of living a long life as this is a major key in attaining happiness. Surely, happiness is an important factor in eliminating stress and decreasing cortisol levels.

Unfortunately, if you are constantly under stress, the high cortisol levels will make it more difficult to lose inches from your waistline. Stress is also considered one of the primary underlying causes of heart disease. Many studies have shown that the high levels of cortisol from long-term stress can increase high-density lipoprotein (HDL), triglycerides, blood sugar, and blood pressure.[131] These changes brought on by stress are known to be probable risk factors for heart disease. Stress can promote the buildup of plaque deposits in the arteries and increase the risk of stroke and heart attack. This is why stress reduction is important and should be a priority when seeking reduction in your waistline. Reduction of stress will also help with decreasing inflammation in your body and move you into a good position to minimize your risk of complications from Covid-19.

If you would like to maximize the reduction in the size of your waistline, you will have to accompany your exercise and core work with the anti-inflammatory diet with the keto push. This is a term for a modified anti-inflammatory diet that shifts you to a state of ketosis. This will allow you to maximize the fat loss in your body's midsection.

8
ANTI-INFLAMMATORY DIET WITH KETO PUSH

The keto diet is basically a very low-carbohydrate and higher-fat diet that sets up a state of ketosis in your body. Most people eat simple carbohydrates (rice, bread, pasta and sweets) for a large portion of their diet. As mentioned in Chapter 2, simple carbohydrates are glucogenic. Your body will break down the simple carbohydrates and pass glucose into the bloodstream. This will increase the insulin levels in your blood. Your body will then store fats and keep the fat in your body in case of a shortage of carbohydrates. Because most people continue to eat simple carbohydrates, this glut of glucogenic fuel never happens and the body fat (visceral and subcutaneous) just continues to grow and enlarge your mid-section.

If you fast or deprive your body of simple carbohydrates, the energy for the muscles, organs and brain will have to come from somewhere else. The reduction in simple carbohydrates puts your body into a state of "ketosis," where fat from your body and your diet is burned for energy *(App 8-1 Rec.+)*. Your body produces fuel molecules called "ketones" because the glucose usually formed from the breakdown of simple carbohydrates is scarce. Your body switches its fuel supply to run primarily on fat, actually burning fat 24 hours a day. When your insulin levels are very low, fat burning can increase dramatically. Your liver is able to produce ketones to nourish your muscles and organs, and most importantly your brain. Your brain has high energy requirements and can shift from using glucose to primarily ketones when you are on a keto diet.

One of the primary advantages of the keto diet is the steady supply of energy without the peaks and valleys noted with a high carbohydrate diet. When you eat a lot of simple carbs (glucogenic foods), sugars will flow into your blood and your pancreas will release lots of insulin. The insulin will bring the glucose levels down and eventually you will hit a valley off of the peak and you may feel weaker and tired. This peak and valley from sugar highs and lows will no longer occur if you shift to a ketonic state. By decreasing the need for insulin with the keto diet, your pancreas will work less and this has been shown to help with Type 2 diabetics.[132] In this randomized clinical trial, 263 adults with Type 2 diabetes were placed on a low-carb diet or high-carb, low-fat diet. In the study, the participants on the low-carb diet experienced lowered average blood sugar levels and weight loss at the end of 48 weeks. For those with Type 2 diabetes, the low-carb diet seems to improve average blood sugar levels better in the first year than the high-carbohydrate, low-fat diet. By improving your blood sugar levels you are improving your diabetes and likely lessening your vulnerability to the SARS-CoV-2 virus.

Achieving ketosis

When you fast, you start to use up your glycogen stores and then your body transitions to using fat for energy. Your body fat is then broken down into fatty acids and ketones and a state of ketosis is achieved. You may need to fast for two to four days to achieve ketosis. Obviously, fasting is not desirable and most people do not want to go this route. Additionally, staying in a state of ketosis while fasting for an extended period of time to allow loss of body fat is not realistic. However, short periods of fasting or occasionally skipping meals is a reasonable alternative to lower caloric intake and promote weight loss. On some days when more carbs are consumed, skipping a meal such as lunch will make it easier to stay below the upper carb limit. If longer periods of fasting are instituted, you may experience some muscle loss in addition to fat loss *(App 8-2 Ref.)*. **Shorter periods of fasting will shift you to a ketotic state without risking muscle loss** *(App 8-3 Ref.)*. You should consult with your physician if you plan on any extended period of fasting as this may be problematic if you have existing comorbidities.

To get into a state of ketosis, most will have to eat less than 50 grams of net carbohydrates, measured as total carbs minus fiber, each day. It is very easy to eat over 50 grams of net carbohydrates in a day if you consider a single slice of bread is about 21 net carbs. Even that tasty apple is 25 carbs. So you can readily see that staying below that 50 grams net carbs threshold is difficult. That is why the typical keto diet is composed of 75% fats, 20% protein and 5% carbohydrates. This is significantly different from the typical anti-inflammatory diet. However, you can make modifications to your anti-inflammatory diet to incorporate a keto angle and help lose weight and body fat. A typical keto diet allows you to eat many types of fat that are not anti-inflammatory such as bacon, fatty red meat and prominently high-fat dairy. The high-fat dairy includes; hard cheeses, high-fat cream, butter, etc. The high-fat dairy products are extremely inflammatory and should be excluded from an anti-inflammatory diet. On the other hand, the keto diet and the anti-inflammatory diet have a lot in common. The major common characteristics are cutting simple carbohydrates and increasing fats. The problem is the types of fats as many fats are inflammatory and could potentially promote heart disease.

To go into a state of ketosis on the anti-inflammatory diet you will have to be more selective in your choice of complex carbohydrates. Vegetables such as broccoli, cauliflower, green beans, and asparagus would be good options. Nuts and seeds such as almonds, walnuts and peanuts are also good options for the keto shift. Avocado is the perfect item to add to the diet to provide good fat and almost no carbs. An entire avocado has 2 to 4 grams net carbs depending on the size of the avocado *(App 8-4 AIF +)*. You would like to consume food items that are higher in good fat and low in carbohydrates. This will allow you to get the important calories that you need yet stay below the 50-gram net carb limit per day.

Balancing carbs and fats

To fully understand carbohydrates, you will need to understand what net carbs are. For example, if you eat a cup of broccoli, there are a total of six grams of carbohydrates in that cup. There are also two grams of fiber in that same cup of broccoli. We take the six grams of total carbs and subtract the two grams of fiber leaving you with a net carbs total of four grams. The net carbs in one cup of Romaine lettuce is 0.4, one cup of cauliflower (steamed) is 1.8, kale is 4.2, spinach is 0.2 and green beans is 5.8. As you can see, you can still eat a lot of vegetables and easily stay below the total net carb level of 50 per day.

The tricky part comes with adding some fruit. As mentioned earlier, an apple will add 21 to 25 grams of net carbohydrates. Strawberries are eight grams of net carbs in a cup. One cup of blueberries is about 17 grams of net carbs. Simply having a green tea blueberry shake with the frozen blueberries gives you 20 to 30 grams of net carbs. If you add the apple after dinner that gives you another 20 net carbs (small apple). This puts you over the daily allowance of 50 carbs for the day. It is very difficult to stay under the upper limit of carbs unless you are eating mostly fat throughout the day. However, the blueberries and apple have good anti-inflammatory properties. This is where you will have to weigh the benefits to each diet (anti-inflammatory versus keto). By modifying the proportions of fats, protein and complex carbs, you can still stay anti-inflammatory, decrease total caloric intake and get to a mildly ketotic state.

The key to the anti-inflammatory diet with keto push is altering the proportions of the typical ketogenic diet. Instead of the proportions of 75% fats, 20% protein and 5% carbohydrates of the typical keto diet, the proportions can be modified to 60% fats, 25% protein and 15% complex carbohydrates, give or take here and there. (Figure 14) In this case, you will be replacing some of the fat with more protein and complex carbohydrates. The key is to limit the carbohydrates to only complex carbs (vegetables, lettuces, etc.). **Healthy oils, which are fats (olive oil, avocado oil, etc.), are added to all of the complex carbohydrate portions of the meal.** For example, broccoli, cauliflower,

CHAPTER 8: Anti-inflammatory Diet with Keto Push

asparagus, green beans and kale can be generously covered with extra-virgin olive oil. If the complex carbohydrates are eaten with the good oils, then you are consuming the fats with the complex carbs. This is key and simulates many of the features of the Mediterranean diet. The actual fat component of the keto push will be in the form of good oils and proteins with good oils. That involves eating foods with lots of omega-3 fatty acids such as wild salmon, mackerel, herring, anchovies, sardines, avocado, flax seed, chia seeds, walnuts, etc. *(App 8-5 Ref.)* So simply by making different choices on the proteins and carbs you eat, you can add the good fats and get to the keto push. **The concept is to add good fats in the non-fat portions of your meal.** The keto push also includes taking the omega-3 fish oil supplements. These omega-3 fatty acid supplements can add a significant amount of good fats to your dietary intake. You can also add the balsamic vinegar that will help to allow some of carbs to pass through your system without even being completely absorbed as a sugar. You would like to avoid any empty carbs that do not in some way either have inherently good levels of omega-3 fats or carry those good fats in how they are prepared. The strategy is to think of every food item as a means **to add the good fat** while trying to keep the net carbs less than 50 grams. In essence you are tricking your body to think you are eating a lot of "dirty keto foods" but actually you are eating lots of healthy anti-inflammatory foods with lots of omega-3 fatty acids. This strategy can be very effective and will allow you to get to a mildly ketogenic state while remaining "anti-inflamed."

Everyone is different and how reliably you get into the ketogenic state may vary from person to person. You may have to do some experimentation to determine what foods you must eat to form the necessary ketones to lose the belly fat. You may have to go hard core with virtually no carbs on some days and more balanced fat, protein and carbs on other days. In some cases, you may need to skip a meal (lunch) to stay in the ketonic state. The key is to avoid falling off the wagon and going back to the simple carbs. You will be able to monitor your progress by weighing yourself, measuring your abdominal girth and possibly even measuring your blood ketones or urine ketones.

Measuring ketone levels

When you start the anti-inflammatory diet with the keto push you will note several changes in your body. One of the first changes you will note is that your breath takes on a fruity fragrance or just simply "bad breath." This is due to the elevated levels of ketones, specifically, acetone.[133] After 12 hours on a ketogenic diet, study participants showed a 3.5-fold increase in breath acetone and a 13-fold increase in urinary acetoacetate. The change in your breath indicates that you have shifted to a ketogenic state. While in the ketogenic state, there will be a lowering of glucose levels in your blood and increased ketones such as beta-hydroxybutyrate (BHB).

Measuring your blood ketone levels is the most precise means of determining if you in a ketogenic state. You can accomplish this using a "home use" ketone meter that measures blood ketones with a drop of blood from a needle stick.[134] You can use a similar self-testing device that does require a finger prick *(App 8-6 Rec.+)*. You can test yourself at least once a week to make sure you are in an optimal nutritional ketosis state. When you are at a non-ketotic state burning carbs, your ketone levels should be less than 0.5 mmol/L *(App 8-7 Rec. +)*. To reach a level of nutritional ketosis due to your ketogenic diet, you will need to get to 0.5 mmol/L or higher. You are at a light nutritional ketosis, if your ketone level is between 0.5 mmol/L and 1.0 mmol/L. The optimal range for nutritional ketosis is when your ketone levels are between 1.0 mmol/L and 3.0 mmol/L. After exercising while on a keto diet your ketone levels peak out at 3mmol/L to 5 mmol/L. While on the anti-inflammatory diet with keto push, you will likely be in the light nutritional ketosis with your ketone level between 1.0 mmol/L and 3.0 mmol/L. This will be adequate to get some of the benefits of the ketotic state, yet keeping low levels of inflammation.

Ketone levels can also be measured in your urine and your breath. You can easily do this by testing your urine for ketones. Acetone breath analyzers and carbon dioxide breath sampling devices can be used but are not as accurate as the blood measurements *(App 8-8 Rec.)*. It is very easy to measure ketone levels in your urine with test strips. If you are averse to sticking yourself then you can stick to the urine testing. Most do not monitor because they know when they are in the ketogenic state, noting the many changes as they transition to the fat burning state of metabolism.

Side effects of a keto diet

If you are ketogenic you will also note weight loss and soon after that some fat loss. The initial loss of weight may be related to burning stored carbs and water *(App 8-9 Ref. +)*. This will be followed by loss of stored fat as long as you remain on the diet and are in a caloric deficit. In other words, as long as you are burning more calories than you are taking in, you will lose weight. You may also note a decreased appetite while on the ketogenic diet. The ketones themselves may directly affect your brain to decrease your appetite.[135]

When you adopt a keto diet, your body will be burning fat instead of carbs. This will create a shift in the fuel for your brain. Your brain will work more efficiently on the ketones. However, when you first start the keto diet you may experience "keto flu" with symptoms of "brain fog" and lethargy *(App 8-10 Ref.)*. This period of lethargy and low energy is due to the shift from burning carbs to a fat burning fuel source. This can take weeks to start to feel good. Be sure you stick it out. You should take the electrolyte-enhanced fluids during this time period and continue the electrolytes while on the diet *(App 8-11 Ref.)*. When this period of brain fog occurs, you know that you are starting to enter the keto push. These symptoms or tiredness and fogginess will be short-lived in most people and you will then experience improved brain function and increased clarity. Along with the tiredness may be some problems with insomnia. This will eventually be replaced with improved sleep as you settle into the keto push.

You may also experience some digestive issues such as diarrhea or constipation. This is particularly problematic if you go to the "dirty keto" diet with lots of fatty meats and fatty foods. If you are on the anti-inflammatory diet with the keto push, the many complex carbohydrates that you will be eating will help with the constipation issues. This is one of the major advantages of the anti-inflammatory diet with keto push over the more typical high-fat very low-carb keto diet.

As you transition into the diet you will note many of the early side effects. If you are transitioning from the anti-inflammatory diet to keto push, then your symptoms will be relatively minor and short-lived. Monitoring your ketones is a good way to make sure you are in the nutritionally valuable level of the keto push. It may preferable to get the blood ketone monitor or at minimum the urine ketone testing strips.

Some believe that apple cider vinegar can help with the ketotic state. When apple cider vinegar is distilled, the process starts by crushing apples and squeezing out the liquid. Bacteria and yeast are then added to the juice, turning it to alcohol. In another step the alcohol is converted to vinegar by acetic-acid forming bacteria. The apple cider vinegar has low net carbs with only 2.2 grams in a cup and only 50 calories and one gram of sugar. So by drinking it you are not increasing your net carb intake by much. However, does it help your keto diet and will it help you lose weight? Studies are variable in what they state. In a 2009 study, 15 milliliters of apple cider vinegar a day helped with mild weight loss and decrease in abdominal fat in obese Japanese subjects.[136] There is not a lot of data that supports the use of apple cider vinegar with the keto diet. There is some evidence that drinking apple cider vinegar can help curb your cravings for carbs *(App 8-12 Ref.)*. It also may help diabetics with their sugar control. If drinking apple cider vinegar can help you kick the carb habit, then it may be a good option. To drink apple cider vinegar, add two to 10 ounces to a cup of warm water and drink it like a tea. You can add lemon, ginger or turmeric to make it more palatable. My preference is to use balsamic vinegar on salads or as a glaze on vegetables and proteins *(App 8-13 Ref.)*. It has many more anti-inflammatory benefits over apple cider vinegar and has total net carbs of only two grams in a teaspoon *(App 8-14 Ref.)*.

There is the potential for weight loss with the keto diet.[137] Unlike diets focusing on reducing calories, the keto diet helps you lose weight by putting your body into ketosis. While in a ketotic state, your body produces ketones for energy to nourish your organs and your brain. Because your body steadily burns fat as a fuel source, you will start to shed body fat and potentially lose weight. Your body type as well as some hereditary factors will determine how effective the weight loss will be while on the keto diet. While on the anti-inflammatory diet with keto push you will be more likely to lose weight because you are not eating a dirty keto diet and you are also likely eating fewer calories. This is a major advantage of this diet over the typical keto diet.

One of the big problems with the dirty keto diet is how the increased fat intake will affect your blood cholesterol and cardiac status. Increasing your intake of saturated fats can increase your risk of cardiovascular disease.[138] This is a big problem with the dirty keto diet. You may be losing body fat and in the meantime increasing your long-term cardiac risk by eating saturated fats *(App 8-15 Ref.+)*. You can minimize this risk by eating unsaturated fats, particularly polyunsaturated fats. You would like to avoid the "dirty keto" food items such as bacon, chicken wings and processed foods such as sausages and processed deli meats.

Instead of the dirty keto you can consume anti-inflammatory proteins such as skinless chicken breast (free-range organic), lean red meats (grass fed) and wild salmon. Sardines and mackerel are healthy fish that are very high in omega-3 fatty acids. Another fat in the keto/anti-inflammatory diet is fat from olive oil. Extra-virgin olive oil can be added to most of your foods, including salads, shakes and vegetables. It is actually a good idea to drink a couple tablespoons of extra-virgin olive oil a day, as suggested in Chapter 4. Some clinical studies suggest that drinking about two tablespoons (23 grams) of olive oil daily may help to reduce the risk of coronary heart disease due to the monounsaturated fat in olive oil *(App 8-16 Ref.)*. The problem with drinking olive oil is that there are 119 calories in a tablespoon. It is difficult to drink olive oil straight up so I prefer to add it to my green tea shake with blueberries. You can also drizzle extra-virgin olive oil on your other foods.

Obviously avocado is an important component to the keto push. You can include the avocado in your shake, in your salad and with your dinner. You can also drink some avocado oil or add some to your shake or drinks. Avocado can be added to your diet in many different ways. You could start your day with avocado slices on a keto-friendly bread option. Avocados are ready to eat when they are slightly soft and compressible *(App 8-17 Ref.)*. The problem with avocados is that you may have to keep visiting the grocer to have ripe avocados on hand. You can always have ripe avocados if you purchase a bunch and freeze them once they are ripe. You will have to cut the avocados in halves, seed them, wrap with plastic wrap and freeze. You can thaw the avocado half when you are ready to eat it. There are keto-friendly bread options that are made of a combination of apple cider vinegar, organic egg whites, baking powder, salt and water plus the fiber sources of almond flour, golden flax seed and psyllium husk *(App 8-18 Rec.)*. There are two net carbs per slice of this keto-friendly bread. Avocado can also be eaten in everyone's favorite guacamole that is nightshade free *(App 8-19 AIF+)*.

The keto diet is an excellent companion to any efforts to decrease your abdominal fat and achieve that trim waistline that you desire. The combination of the keto state and core exercises is perfect to make the most significant changes to your body and general health. The core exercises will help to tone your muscles and the keto component of the diet will help to lose the fat that would otherwise hide your defined abs *(App 8-20 Rec. Video +)*.

As with any diet, particularly the keto diet, you should consult with your physician prior to embarking on it. This is particularly important if you have other medical comorbidities such as diabetes, hypertension or heart disease. Your physician will note your medical history and determine if you are a good candidate for the anti-inflammatory diet with keto push. Your physician is more likely to approve of you starting the anti-inflammatory diet with keto push versus the typical dirty keto diet.

There are many supplements that may help to keep you in the ketogenic state, but there are few if any reputable studies verifying safety or efficacy. Some safe supplements to take with your keto push include magnesium, omega-3 fatty acids, vitamin D and minerals *(App 8-21 Ref.)*. When you transition to a keto diet you may experience keto flu with symptoms such as headache, muscle cramps and fatigue.[139] Adding foods that are rich in sodium, magnesium and potassium can help to prevent these symptoms. Dark leafy greens such as kale, purple romaine, nuts, avocados and seeds are all keto-friendly foods that are high in both magnesium and potassium. Electrolyte supplements containing sodium, potassium and magnesium are available as well *(App 8-22 Rec.)*. Some of these supplements may help promote the ketotic state; however, you should consult with your physician before taking such supplements. The key supplement will be the omega-3 fatty acids in the capsule form. This supplement will provide the important omega-3 fatty acids as well as help you add the good fats to your diet to become ketotic.

Carb consumption and anxiety

There is a distinct association between carbohydrate consumption and anxiety.[140] Individuals with elevated blood sugar levels are more than two-times more likely to develop depressive illness. Elevated HbA1c is a well-established risk factor for dementia and is now considered a risk factor for depression, ADHD, anxiety, bipolar disorder and other mood disturbances. The mechanisms of action may be due to oxidative damage affecting nerve function in the brain through elevated insulin levels and increased inflammation and hypoglycemia. Those on the ketogenic diet state they feel more like themselves with less anxiety. This may be directly related to ketone bodies crossing the blood-brain barrier and influencing neurotransmitters.

The ketogenic diet has been shown to reduce overactivity of the nervous system and potentially help those with seizure disorders.[141] With the ketogenic diet there is a shift in the energy metabolism from glycolytic energy production to energy generation through oxidative phosphorylation (fatty acid b-oxidation and ketone-body production). This change in how energy is produced is part of the anticonvulsant mechanism of the ketogenic diet.[142] Through a similar mechanism, the ketogenic diet has been shown to regulate mood and reduce excitatory neurotransmitter excess to reduce anxiety and stress response.[143] The expression of gamma aminobutyric acid (GABA) is increased when ketones cross the blood-brain barrier. GABA is a neuro-inhibitory amino acid that mellows out the brain and body. Low levels of GABA in the brain can drive irritability, impulse control issues, compulsive eating, cravings and uncontrolled racing thoughts. Increasing GABA expression with the use of dietary ketosis can stabilize moods and reduce anxiety *(App 8-23 Rec.+)*. By lowering your glucose level and reducing insulin response, the ketogenic diet may further improve your mood and reduce excitatory neuron activity.

The combination of the anti-inflammatory diet and the ketogenic diet can have great impact on brain function. Inflammation is mediated by chemical compounds such as prostaglandins, leukotrienes, and interleukins that are released in excess in response to eating inflammatory foods. These inflammatory chemical responders can cross the blood-brain barrier and directly interfere with neurotransmitter signaling, brain function and mood stability.[144] Additionally, inflammatory chemicals in the digestive tract can stimulate the sympathetic nervous system to initiate "fight or flight" signaling and increase anxiety and stress.[145] When you eat inflammatory or glucogenic foods, your body responds with these fight or flight signals with a generalized state of unease and elevated levels of anxiety.

The anti-inflammatory diet with the keto push can reduce inflammation, enhance neurotransmitter function and reduce stress response, alleviating the chronic fight or flight worried mode that can drive depression, anxiety and panic. This combination diet can potentially do much more than just flatten your stomach. If you are calm and less stressed, this can surely help your relationships and potentially extend your lifespan. This in itself is a good reason to embark on the anti-inflammatory diet with keto push. A shortened name for the anti-inflammatory diet with keto-push is the AI-keto (eye·key·toe) diet.

9

EFFECTS OF ANTI-INFLAMMATORY DIET ON YOUR SKIN AND AGING

Skin aging occurs through two distinct processes; intrinsic aging and extrinsic aging.[146] Intrinsic aging is the same process that ages all of the organs in your body and represents chronological aging. Extrinsic aging is influenced by external factors such as sun exposure and ultraviolet radiation. (Figure 15) Other environmental factors such as pollution and a dry climate can influence extrinsic aging. Smoking, sleep deprivation and an inflammatory diet can significantly affect skin aging as well. Genetic influence on skin aging is part of the equation as Caucasians have an earlier onset of skin wrinkling and sagging of tissues than Asian and other darker-skinned ethnicities.[147] Therefore, if you have darker, more sebaceous skin you will likely see slower skin aging notwithstanding your external and environmental factors. European skin types are more likely to see earlier skin aging for multiple reasons, including less sebaceous activity and less facial fat.

The amount of facial fat in your skin is a critical factor in skin aging. In youth, fat in the face is evenly distributed, with areas of extra fat that plump up the cheeks, temples in the forehead and areas around the eyes and mouth. With aging, facial fat atrophies and redistributes lower in the face resulting in sagging skin, tired looking eyes, sagging jowls and extra neck skin. (Figure 16) This general loss of facial fat contributes greatly to facial aging and is definitely more prominent in Caucasian ethnicities over East Asian populations. When we rejuvenate the face, we can inject facial fillers or the patient's own fat into deficient areas of the face. By plumping up the face we can replace the atrophied fat and create a more youthful, full facial appearance. These fat loss changes are not necessarily something that you can control with your diet. However, many of the other factors such as skin wrinkling and skin hydration can be controlled by avoiding sun exposure and staying well hydrated.

One of the drawbacks to going on this diet is that you may lose weight—and a consequence of the weight loss is that you may lose fat in your face and the tissues may droop a bit more. This can be a bigger problem for Caucasians who have a greater tendency to lose fat in their faces with weight loss. If you choose to go on the keto push diet, then you may lose even more facial fat.

UV radiation

Exposed areas of the body such as the face and neck suffer the most from the influence of extrinsic factors such as UV irradiation. Excessive exposure of these regions may result in premature skin aging and formation of benign skin lesions such as actinic keratosis and malignant skin tumors such as basal cell carcinoma, squamous cell carcinoma and malignant melanoma.[148] These disease processes are initiated by free radical damage to the skin, where an extra electron is stolen from other molecules in the body. When these molecules are taken away, it causes direct damage to our skin's DNA, which results in accelerated skin aging and potential formation of skin cancers. Over time, the effects of free radical damage often become more and more noticeable. Mitochondrial DNA mutations and protein oxidation can disrupt the defense against protein macromolecular damage and apoptosis induction. In non-exposed areas such as the inner side of the upper arm, aging is mainly attributed to intrinsic factors such as genetic predisposition.

One of the most important long-term means to keep your skin looking good is to avoid sun exposure. UV radiation can severely damage the extrinsic components of the skin and create skin wrinkling and sun spots and irregular pigmentation of your skin. These changes are "etched" into your skin and are difficult to completely remove. With invasive and minimally invasive methods the extrinsic skin can be improved, but this requires time and money. You should try your best to limit sun exposure and use sunscreen all the time. Apply a moisturizer containing sunscreen daily, if possible. There are many options for sunscreens, and this can be confusing. It is best to use a sunscreen that has broad spectrum protection against UVA and UVB rays and is PABA free with an SPF of 30 or higher *(App 9-1 Ref.+)*. It is a good idea to wear a wide- brimmed hat whenever possible. When you are on the water there is a lot of reflected sunlight so you must reapply the sunscreen frequently. Chronic sun exposure is very damaging to your skin and should be avoided at all cost.

Hydration

Staying hydrated is also very important to the health and appearance of your skin. When you drink a glass of water, it does not necessarily go directly toward improving the appearance of your skin. However, staying hydrated is important to normal bodily functions and also prevents dehydration. We know that dehydration can result in a loss of skin elasticity.[149] Staying hydrated also helps to clear toxins from your body that can negatively affect your skin and other organs in your body. You will definitely want to avoid becoming dehydrated. Unfortunately, many people are chronically dehydrated because they do not drink enough water to account for the amount of diuresis that occurs in response to coffee and alcohol intake during the day. Most would agree that you should drink eight glasses of water a day. Coffee, tea and alcohol will make you urinate, and this will tend to dehydrate you. If you have coffee or tea you should add a couple more glasses of water to counteract the dehydrating effect.

You should drink water with electrolytes if you are drinking a lot of water to rehydrate after becoming dehydrated. This is particularly important if you have experienced a bout of diarrhea after a gastrointestinal problem (food poisoning, flu, etc.) In these cases you will have lost some electrolytes and minerals and will need to replenish these nutrients. If you only replace it with water you could potentially become hyponatremic (low blood sodium levels) or lose other important electrolytes. This can be seen in marathon runners who sweat a lot during a race and drink just water as a replacement. You can add an electrolyte balance replacement product minus the carbohydrates (sugars) typically found in sports drinks. There are several very good electrolyte replacement products that you can add to your water to replace lost electrolytes *(App 9-2 Rec.)*. You can add the electrolyte replacement to one in every three glasses of water to make sure you get the electrolytes needed to stay balanced as well as hydrated.

If you frequently fly on an airplane, your skin will get extra ultraviolet exposure and your skin will get dried out. The airplane cabins tend to have very low humidity and will really dry out your skin. You should apply sunscreen before getting on a plane and also stay hydrated by drinking a lot of water. Many people will drink alcohol and coffee on a plane and this will tend to further dehydrate you. You can have one glass of wine and then spend the rest of the time trying to rehydrate. You should try to avoid any coffee or tea and limit the alcohol. It is also a good idea to apply a good moisturizer when you take longer flights.

Diet

Seemingly unrelated skin conditions such as acne, rosacea, skin wrinkles, psoriasis and large pores are clearly linked to inflammation. One of the best ways to slow the effects of aging on your skin is to begin an anti-inflammatory diet *(App 9-3 Rec.+)*. Nicolas Perricone is one of the most prominent doctors who has promoted the anti-inflammatory diet for aging skin *(App 9-4 Ref.)*. He promotes a three-pronged approach that starts with the anti-inflammatory diet and follows with inflammation reducing supplements. The third component involves topical treatments such as creams with alpha-lipoic acid (ALA). I have seen many patients improve the quality and appearance of their skin with the institution of the anti-inflammatory diet. Patients themselves have seen dramatic improvements, and the anti-aging effects are well documented.[150]

Acne has been linked to a high-glycemic diet, which is high in carbohydrates and has a high rate of carbohydrate absorption. Foods with a high GI—such as sugar, white rice, white bread and pasta—are rapidly absorbed, leading to higher serum sugar (glucose) levels and corresponding elevated levels of insulin. Insulin and IGF-1 have been shown to increase skin oil production, increase androgen hormone (male hormone), and increase androgen availability, which contribute to the development of acne.[151] If you cut sugars and simple carbohydrates from your diet, you can dramatically improve your acne. Your acne can be improved to an even greater extent if you go full bore on the anti-inflammatory diet and take the green tea and supplements as well. The same applies for patients with rosacea and psoriasis as these are inflammation driven disorders.

Rosacea is a chronic skin condition that results in redness of the skin of the cheeks, chin, nose and forehead. It affects over 14 million Americans (one in 20 people). It can present as a red bulbous shape to the nose and can progress to a more serious issue: rhinophyma. Rosacea shares genetic risk loci with autoimmune diseases such as Type 1 diabetes mellitus (T1DM), rheumatoid arthritis and celiac disease. The association between autoimmune disorders and rosacea suggests it has an underlying autoimmune etiology. Many of my patients who have rosacea saw significant improvement in their symptoms with strict adherence to an anti-inflammatory diet. Omega-3 fatty acids have shown to improve symptoms in patients with rosacea and stress and alcohol worsened symptoms.[152]

Systemic lupus erythematosus (SLE), or lupus, is thought to be similar to rosacea, and symptoms have been improved with an anti-inflammatory diet. Lupus is an autoimmune disease where the body's immune system attacks normal healthy tissue such as the skin, joints and other organs. Patients with lupus can improve their symptoms by going on an anti-inflammatory diet.[153]

You can assess overall health by looking at a person's skin. People who are healthy tend to have vibrant skin with good skin tone. Patients with multiple comorbidities tend to have poorly vascularized skin with poor skin tone and more acne-like imperfections. Once your skin starts to reflect your underlying health, you may be progressing to a stage of severe chronic disease. You should never let yourself reach that stage.

10 ARTHRITIS, BACK PAIN AND THE ANTI-INFLAMMATORY DIET

The anti-inflammatory diet can have a tremendous impact on the status of your back and joints. Back pain comes in many different forms. The two major categories include mechanical versus inflammatory back pain. Mechanical back pain is related to some disruption in the proper alignment or workings of the spine, muscles, nerves and intervertebral disks. This type of back pain may occur with overdoing a workout, moving in the incorrect manner, falling awkwardly or just sleeping in the incorrect position. The other type of back pain is inflammatory in origin and is called ankylosing spondylitis or axial spondylarthritis *(App 10-1 Ref.)*. Inflammatory back pain (IBP) is a condition of pain localized to the axial spine and sacroiliac joints or lower back and is more of a chronic process. Inflammatory back pain typically presents as stiffness, pain and decreased range of motion. This disorder typically starts at a younger age (typically under 35) and lasts for three months or more. The pain is more intense in the morning or with inactivity and gets better as you increase activity and exercise. The pain can start in the lower back and radiate to the buttocks. Non-steroidal anti-inflammatory agents are very effective in treating inflammatory back pain. With inflammatory back pain you may also experience other symptoms that may seem unrelated, including eye inflammation, inflammatory bowel disease, psoriasis or pain in your peripheral joints such as your ankles or knees.

The above symptoms of inflammatory back pain, in addition to evidence of damage to the sacroiliac joints or the presence of the genetic marker HLA-B27 on a blood test, may confirm the diagnosis of ankylosing spondylitis.[154] You will have to see your doctor or a rheumatologist to get confirmation of the diagnosis.

Rheumatoid arthritis is a disease that involves your own immune system mistakenly attacking your joints, causing pain, swelling and stiffness. If left untreated, rheumatoid arthritis can cause permanent damage to your joints. This chronic disease can affect the eyes, skin, lung, kidneys, heart and blood vessels as well. Over time, rheumatoid arthritis can deform joints and cause severe damage to organs. Rheumatoid arthritis can present in many different ways but early symptoms can include fatigue, weight loss, joint tenderness and pain as well as joint swelling. Risk factors for developing RA include your sex and age, with women more likely to develop it in middle age. Family history puts you at increased risk as well. Environmental factors and obesity are also thought to be risk factors to develop RA. Rheumatoid arthritis occurs at an incidence of approximately three cases per 10,000 people. However, the incidence is increasing due to unknown reasons.

Ankylosing spondylitis and rheumatoid arthritis are chronic progressive inflammatory diseases, leading to joint damage. However, their etiology and symptomatology are different and are treated differently. Ankylosing spondylitis can progress over time to cause fusion of the vertebrae leaving you in stooped posture as well as other long-term consequences. Rheumatoid arthritis can progress to deform the joints and cause organ damage. One thing they have in common are the inflammatory component of the diseases. Reducing inflammation can be helpful in reducing pain and potentially slow the progression of these diseases *(App 10-2 Ref.)*.[155] There is conflicting data on whether diet can actually slow the progression of the diseases. However, it is clear that the symptoms can be improved significantly if you avoid inflammatory foods. **By decreasing your body's inflammation the pain associated with the inflamed joints will likely decrease.**

Tendonitis is a disorder that involves inflammation of the tendons that connect bones to muscles. It can affect the wrist, elbow, fingers, thigh and ankle as well as other parts of the body. It can occur from injuring the tendon during sports, working out or simply by moving incorrectly. Tennis elbow is a typical form of tendonitis. Inflammation of the tendons can become a chronic problem in some, particularly when the tendon is constantly being used. Most forms of tendinitis can be improved by rest, physical therapy and pain medication. However, some of us are unable to completely rest the tendon and the inflammation can persist for many months or years and ultimately result in tendinosis or calcific tendonitis, which can lead to irreversible damage to the tendon. Bursitis is an inflammation of the joint that can occur from overuse or injury as well. Both of these disorders can be dramatically improved by instituting the anti-inflammatory diet and adding anti-inflammatory supplements *(App 10-3 AIF)*.

In my clinical study, patients with chronic inflammatory disorders including inflammatory back pain, tendonitis and rheumatoid arthritis improved significantly on the anti-inflammatory diet. They could associate the consumption of inflammatory foods with increased back and joint pain. The anti-inflammatory diet has been shown to effectively improve symptoms related to inflammatory back pain *(App 10-4 AIF)*. In my experience, patients with mechanical back pain related to more acute forms of back and joint injury also experienced improvement in symptoms of their pain while on the anti-inflammatory diet. There is evidence that an anti-inflammatory diet can improve symptoms related to some forms of vertebral disk disease *(App 10-4 AIF)*. This will require eating lower glycemic index foods and anti-inflammatory foods as described in earlier chapters.

If your back and joint symptoms are improved with taking a non-steroidal anti-inflammatory drug (NSAID), you can consider either replacing it or adding the anti-inflammatory diet.[156] Non-steroidal anti-inflammatory drugs (NSAIDs) can have significant side effects, including gastrointestinal ulcers and bleeding, cardiovascular events such as hypertension and heart failure, kidney damage and platelet dysfunction.[157] You have many options other than NSAIDs for treating the pain associated with inflammatory disorders. At the top of the list are omega-3 fatty acids, green tea and curcumin *(App 10-5 Rec.+)*. The omega-3 fatty acids can be added to your diet through foods such as salmon, sardines, mackerel, flax seed, etc. You could also take omega-3 fatty acid capsules as discussed in Chapter 5. Incorporating turmeric to your

CHAPTER 10: Arthritis, Back Pain and the Anti-inflammatory Diet   109

meal preparation will add you some curcumin in your diet. You can take a curcumin supplement that will decrease inflammation as well *(App 10-6 Rec.+)*. If you take curcumin, you should take a form that has pepper or its equivalent to improve absorption of the active compound. If you are able to decrease the amount of NSAIDs that you consume for your body pains, that would be an important first step in decreasing the likelihood of getting a complication from the use of these medications.

It is evident that most forms of inflammatory back and joint pain can be improved on the anti-inflammatory diet and anti-inflammatory supplements. Many forms of mechanical back and joint pain can be improved as well. You can easily assess this for yourself by noting the consumption of inflammatory foods and your subsequent experience with back or joint pain. If you eat a pizza with ice cream, are you more sore and uncomfortable the next morning? On the other hand, if you are on a strict anti-inflammatory diet, are your symptoms improved? You can test this out for yourself. Fill out a daily journal and record what you eat and drink and also record your symptoms of back pain or joint pain. Also record the amount of NSAIDs or other medications taken to treat the pain. You may be surprised to find that inflammatory foods are associated with increased back and joint pain. You will be able to pinpoint specific types of foods that are the worst when it comes to increasing your pain. In either case, adhering to an anti-inflammatory diet will likely improve your overall health and could slow the progression of chronic inflammatory disease or help you heal a mechanical injury to your body's joints. The core exercises and weight loss will be important as well to help move along the recovery. You may want to consider the anti-inflammatory diet with the keto push to lose weight and decrease inflammation. Incorporating the anti-inflammatory diet will surely ease your body pains. You are capable of decreasing your body's inflammation and related painful back and/or joints simply by changing what you eat and drink. It's time to make a change and get off of the potentially harmful medications.

11 PRACTICAL WAYS TO INCORPORATE THE ANTI-INFLAMMATORY DIET

It can be very difficult to incorporate an anti-inflammatory diet into your daily routine because we are all very busy and have little time to spend cooking up special meals or creating anti-inflammatory options. In this chapter I will go into some strategies to incorporate the anti-inflammatory diet into your life.

Meal planning

There are several ways to practically incorporate this type of diet into your daily routine. A good start is to write out a plan for your upcoming week of meals on a day-by-day basis. This way you can shop for what you need and save time during the work week. It is also helpful to fall back on some staples that you can always rely on in a pinch. A good example would be a hearty salad with baby greens and balsamic vinegar and olive oil dressing. For your protein you can use chicken, low mercury tuna, hard-boiled-eggs, and nuts. You can include some avocado to add calories and to give you the fat to make you feel satisfied. You can eat such a salad for any lunch or dinner and add an almond butter sandwich on Ezekiel bread or some baby carrots with hummus. You could also have a protein shake as a meal anytime during the day. Other quick options include avocado toast on Ezekiel bread or deli turkey on Ezekiel bread with lettuce and an avocado spread instead of mayo. If you are on the keto push you will need to be more selective in the proteins and carbs that you eat as discussed earlier.

As you set up the list of meals during the week, you should think about making a larger portion size so some of the leftovers can be eaten another day that week. A good option is to cook a couple of spatchcock chickens. Eat a portion of one chicken and refrigerate the remainder. Another good option is to cook several chicken breasts and keep the leftovers for subsequent meals or for lunch salads. The key is to have a good protein source that will last four or five days.

For the meal plan, you can have a couple of chicken options, a salmon option and a turkey option. I'll sketch out some examples of what a full week on the diet might look like in the next chapter. You can work in a red meat option as long as you use grass-fed organic beef. Avoid any chicken or turkey unless it is free-range organic and not corn fed. Include a vegetable for your complex carbohydrate such as broccoli, cauliflower, asparagus, spinach, edamame (soybean) or green beans. Be sure to add the olive oil when you prepare the vegetables to get the added good fat. You can also add a salad with the meal. **Try to avoid all simple carbohydrates such as bread, rice or potatoes.** This may be one of the most difficult aspects of the anti-inflammatory diet. There are carbohydrate replacements that you can incorporate such as cauliflower rice, cauliflower bread or quinoa. Quinoa is a seed or grain and not a simple carbohydrate. It has anti-inflammatory properties and can be used to replace rice in your diet. Quinoa has a lot of protein, fiber, vitamins and minerals and has a nice nutty flavor. If you are on the keto push you should avoid quinoa.

You can plan a "change of pace" meal once or twice a week so you do not go crazy eating chicken and salmon all of the time. Options include an anti-inflammatory pizza made with a cauliflower crust, chickpea flour crust or almond crust instead of a flour crust (not on keto push). Instead of a tomato-based sauce you can use olive oil with crushed garlic and salt and pepper spread over the surface of the crust. Then add precooked chicken or ground turkey meatballs. Add red peppers, onions or mushrooms as desired. Do not precook the vegetables. You can use artificial cheeses that are soy-based, but most are not very tasty. My preference is to go cheese free and just enjoy the taste of the crust and toppings.

Another change of pace meal could be something made with tofu, which is keto-friendly. Tofu can be very helpful to the anti-inflammatory diet. Some researchers have found that soy food consumption was related to lower circulating levels of IL-

6, TNFα, sTNF-R1 and 2 and pivotal cytokines in the inflammatory cascade, which have been associated with many chronic diseases.[158] You can prepare tofu in many different ways. Using a turmeric-based flavoring, tofu can act as your protein source by itself or in a stir-fry with vegetables. Tofu can also be used in miso soup or in tofu burgers. You can get the burgers premade or make them yourself *(App 11-1 AIF+)*. Tofu can become a major protein sources in your diet without compromising variety in your foods. If you choose tofu while on the keto push, make sure you work in a healthy oil such as olive oil or avocado oil.

Another change of pace meal can include ethnic dishes that incorporate anti-inflammatory foods. Tandoori chicken can be very healthy and anti-inflammatory if you replace the yogurt with coconut milk *(App 11-1 AIF+)*. Look into other turmeric-based dishes for your anti-inflammatory diet such as ginger turmeric turkey meatballs *(App 11-3 AIF+)*. The meatballs can be combined with cauliflower pasta and a garlic olive oil sauce. Other healthy options include some Japanese dishes such as miso soup, miso salmon, grilled miso chicken or spinach and broccoli gomaae (all keto-friendly) *(App 11-4 AIF +)*.

There are also many healthy Mediterranean dishes that are the basis for Andrew Weil's anti-inflammatory diet *(App 11-5 Ref.)*. Great Mediterranean dishes include Mediterranean grain bowls with chicken or tofu, Greek salads and grilled shrimp with vegetables. I believe Dr. Weil's meal plan ideas based on the anti-inflammatory diet are very good and can be accessed in any of his recipe books *(App 11-6 Rec.+)*. Once you are able to prepare these dishes you can mix and match the components to create more tasty dishes that are very healthy.

How to order at restaurants

For many, cooking your own meals may not be practical or possible. But you can still follow the diet if you are unable to cook for yourself. If you frequent restaurants for your meals, there are ways to stay with an anti-inflammatory diet. A lot of it comes down to choices and making adjustments to the choices you make. Most restaurants will have a chicken option on the menu. You should choose a grilled chicken breast with no skin and avoid sauces. A simple grilled chicken breast with garlic or other seasonings will usually be safe. Keep in mind that most restaurants use a lot of butter on their foods, particularly if the chicken is sautéed. You can ask for olive oil instead of butter on your meal. The same applies to other meats and fish. Most grilled fish options will be fine, and you can have them put the sauce on the side or just pass on the sauce. Obviously, this will be a bit blander without the sauce, but this is the sacrifice you can make when eating out to make sure you are staying anti-inflammatory. A baked half chicken is usually a good option as well. In this case, take off the skin when you are served the entrée. The skin on the chicken contains all of the saturated fat and is very unhealthy and inflammatory. Avoid chicken wings as these tend to be high calorie, very high in saturated fat and heavily covered with inflammatory additives. You may think you are eating healthy because it is chicken, but it is actually more inflammatory than a piece of lean red meat. If you are on the keto push you can order a chicken leg option as it has more fat but only a little more saturated fat compared to the breast meat.

What about pork, the other white meat? **Unfortunately, pork is inflammatory. The average omega-6 to 3 ratios from pork chops, ground pork and pork tenderloin is 24 to 1**. A high omega-6 to omega-3 fatty acid ratio is highly inflammatory and is to be avoided. It is important to note that this fat content will depend on the specific cut of meat. For example, pork belly may have over 50 grams of fat while leaner cuts of tenderloin could have less than 5g per 100 grams *(App 11-7 Ref.)*. The high omega-6 in pork applies to fatty cuts of pork like bacon and belly pork (more than 5g of omega-6 fatty acids per 100 grams). Leaner cuts of pork like some tenderloin cuts may contain minimal levels of omega-6 (<500 mg per 100 grams). Additionally, many pork products like bacon may contain nitrates, which are associated with gastric and colon cancer.[159] These are good reasons to avoid bacon and processed meats. You can order a lean cut of pork, but try to have it prepared without a sauce or gravy. You will note that the leaner the cut, the less tasty the meat is because the fat gives the meat the flavoring.

When you are ordering sides at a restaurant, choose a complex carbohydrate such as broccoli, cauliflower, asparagus or green beans. You can order these grilled or sautéed in olive oil. Avoid cheesy broccoli or other sides with added cheese. Simple steamed vegetables are less tasty but very healthy. Boiling vegetables can remove a lot of their nutrients. If there is a quinoa or whole wheat couscous option instead of rice, that is a good choice. Avoid choices such as sides of pasta, macaroni and cheese or rice. Things such as French fries, baked potatoes and mashed potatoes should be avoided because they are inflammatory, empty food options. If you would like another side with your meal, consider a side salad or an appetizer. Most restaurants will have some good appetizer choices that are anti-inflammatory. Some good options are grilled octopus, edamame, smoked salmon or some soups. Soups are tricky because most have some inflammatory additives. Miso soup is relatively safe as it is a soup made from fermented soybeans and is not tomato-based. Any soup with dairy is inflammatory and should be avoided. You can always ask the server what ingredients the soup contains.

If you are eating at a restaurant, you should avoid having dessert unless there is a fresh fruit or berry option with no added sugar. In general, desserts have sugar and sugars are inflammatory. Some of the worst desserts are loaded with sugar and fat *(App 11-8 Ref.)*. The Cheesecake Factory has a "warm apple crisp" that has 980 calories, 34g fat (20g saturated fat, 0.5g trans fat), 510mg sodium, 163g carbs (132g sugar, 10g fiber, 10g protein). This is a tremendous amount of sugar and is loaded with saturated fats. This should be a definite pass. At P.F Chang's, the "great wall of chocolate" has 1,700 calories, 71g fat (30g saturated fat, 0g trans fat), 1,410mg sodium, 259g carbs (14 g fiber, 190 g sugar, 17 g protein). You get the picture. If you eat out or carry out, take a look at the nutritional information before you make your choices. Make sure you pass on the high-calorie options. Some healthier options for desserts include grilled fruits, berries, dark chocolates, dark chocolate dipped fruits or biscotti.

If you have a sugar, it is preferable to have a naturally occurring sugar in a fruit such as an apple, melon or berries. Many people will share a dessert at a meal. If you choose to do this just take a taste and leave it at that. This is where your willpower is important.

Alcohol and the anti-inflammatory diet

The big issue when eating out is the alcohol that most will imbibe during a meal. Alcohol is a sugar, and your body treats it as a sugar. Whether you consume wine, beer or a cocktail it is all sugar. Your body is unable to distinguish between the different types of alcohol as it is all processed the same in your gut. **Even alcohol in moderation can cause chronic disease, cancer and contributes to memory loss.**[160] Alcohol intake increases levels of C-reactive protein (CRP) which is a marker for inflammation. On the other hand, red wine may have some anti-inflammatory properties due to its higher concentrations of polyphenols such as resveratrol *(App 11-9 Ref.)*. There are approximately 1.5mg to 13mg of resveratrol per liter of red wine and to gain the beneficial effect you would have to consume 150mg per day or more than 11 liters of wine per day. Therefore, the benefits of the red wine are likely overcome by the effects of the sugars on your system. Despite this nominal benefit, most doctors will tell you that moderate alcohol intake is OK and will not harm you. Moderate alcohol intake may reduce some inflammatory biomarkers such as interleukin-6 and TNF-alpha receptor 2. If you are on the keto push, you should avoid all alcoholic beverages.

The Mediterranean diet incorporates moderate amounts of red wine, and most would agree this diet is generally anti-inflammatory. This creates a dilemma. Where does red wine fit into the scheme of an anti-inflammatory diet? My thoughts are that there may be some small benefit to the red wine that we just are not aware of. However, alcohol intake can have other effects on the body that may not be so helpful. For example, alcohol intake can cause problems with sleep patterns, contribute to dehydration, and result in weight gain. **A study where the participants did not drink for a month noted that 71% slept better; 67% had more energy; 58% lost weight; 57% had better concentration; and 54% had better skin.**[161] When you consume alcohol, portions and types of alcohol matter. According to the National Institute on Alcohol Abuse and Alcoholism, a "standard" alcoholic beverage is defined as; 12 ounces (355 milliliters) of regular beer; eight to nine ounces (237 to 266 milliliters) of malt liquor; five ounces (148 milliliters) of unfortified wine; and 1.5 ounces (44 milliliters) of 80-proof hard liquor *(App 11-10 Ref.)*. When choosing your drink, the least inflammatory options are red wine, tequila, brandy, hard cider, cognac and rum because they tend to be grain free *(App 11-10 Ref.)*. Stay away from sugary or sweet drinks as these tend to be highly inflammatory. If you are on the keto push, pure alcohol products like rum, vodka, gin, tequila and whiskey all contain no carbs and are acceptable.

Studies have shown that alcohol will help the healthy individual fall asleep faster but also reduces REM (rapid eye movement)sleep. In the first half of the night, when the body is metabolizing alcohol, people spend more time in deep, slow-wave sleep and less time in REM sleep.[162] REM sleep decreases in the first half of the night under the influence of alcohol, but is important for memory, emotional stability and mental restoration. During the second half of the night, sleep becomes more actively disrupted. As alcohol is metabolized and any of its sedative effects wear off, the body undergoes a rebound effect. The rebound effect involves a transition from deeper to lighter sleep, with more frequent awakenings during the rest of the night. These awakenings may be very brief and you may not even remember, but the disruptions still interrupt the quality of sleep. During the second half of the night, sleep architecture transitions away from normal, with less time spent in slow wave sleep. Loss of normal sleep architecture can also result in worsening of snoring and sleep disorders. These abnormal changes in sleep can negatively affect circadian rhythms and result in next day tiredness, fatigue, irritability, and difficulty concentrating. Your mood can be negatively affected as well.

With the coronavirus pandemic, many people were drinking more alcoholic beverages. Alcohol sales were up over 50% according to Nielsen during the Covid-19 pandemic *(App 11-12 Ref.)*. This is very problematic, and we will likely see a delayed effect with increased alcohol abuse and alcohol-related diseases. Additionally, alcohol intake can make you more vulnerable to respiratory diseases, including Covid-19. "Alcohol consumption is associated with a range of communicable and non-communicable diseases and mental health disorders, which can make a person more vulnerable to infection by SARS-CoV-2. In particular, alcohol compromises the body's immune system and increases the risk of adverse health outcomes," the WHO (World Health Organization) stated *(App 11-13 Ref.)*. Alcohol's effects on the immune system are broad and act to dampen the body's response to infectious agents and make someone more prone to infection.[163] Alcohol consumption can reduce the number of monocytes and white blood cells that otherwise would fight off disease such as SARS-CoV-2 virus many hours after alcohol consumption.[164]

The increase in alcohol consumption is likely due to a combination of things, including isolation, mood swings and depression. The efficiency of the lungs is compromised with alcohol intake as well, which could compromise one's ability to fight off the SARS-CoV-2 virus.[165] Alcohol can affect the lungs' ability to clear secretions, to cough and to clear viruses. The potential detrimental effects of alcohol are numerous. Even if you drink in moderation, alcohol can have significant lasting effects on your liver and other organs. Alcohol intake can have a detrimental effect on the comorbidities that increase your risk of a bad outcome if you contract Covid-19. Beyond the effects on the immune system, you may accelerate worsening of diabetes and hypertension.[166] Alcohol intake in moderation can also make you dehydrated and can contribute to sleep disorders.

If you decide to have an occasional alcoholic beverage, you should be strategic about when you choose to do so. For example, if you have an important event the following day, it may be wise to avoid drinking alcohol to allow you to feel your best. Also make sure you have only a minimal amount of alcohol. Remember, alcohol is inflammatory and the more you consume the more inflammatory the effect. You could have a half glass of wine instead of the entire glass. This will allow you to get the pleasure of drinking the wine with less of the inflammatory effect. If you only drink occasionally, then it will be easier to avoid alcohol on the off days. This is a very important factor and will dramatically improve your ability to adhere to the diet. I know of many patients who are very good on the anti-inflammatory diet. Their only weakness is the alcohol intake. They want to keep the alcohol in their diet. I tell them just to use common sense when choosing how often they imbibe, what type of alcohol they consume, and how much they drink. It is very interesting when these patients record their progress and symptoms on a daily basis as they find that their symptoms are almost universally worse the day after they drink alcohol.

Takeout and fast food

If you are considering ordering takeout food, there are several ways to keep the options as anti-inflammatory as possible. First of all, it is important to avoid fried foods as these tend to be higher in saturated fats and are also much more inflammatory. Unfortunately, most of the fast food options are fried or higher in saturated fats. For example, even a chicken sandwich at most fast food restaurants is fried or covered with a mayonnaise-based sauce to add flavor. If you would like to have a chicken sandwich, ask them to hold off on the sauce and just eat the chicken breast. Or bring the sandwich home and take the breast and put it on some Ezekiel bread and add avocado or hummus. Pass on the French fries. Another option is to order a sandwich from Panera or Subway. When ordering from these establishments, choose the multigrain option for the bread with turkey or chicken. At some establishments you can also order a "skinny" bread, where they remove some of the bread to decrease the carbohydrates *(App 11-14 Rec.)*. Some establishments have a lettuce wrap option with no bread and just meat wrapped in lettuce. Try to avoid any cheese or processed meats such as salami, pastrami and sausages. Also try to avoid the ham option as this can be higher in saturated fats. You can add lettuce and olives but avoid the tomato. Minimize the application of condiments such as ketchup, mayonnaise or butter. Mustards are fine as long as they do not contain sugar. Unfortunately, many do, so it may be best to stick to the olive oil dressing options for additives.

Some fast food restaurants are trying to add healthier options to choose from. Some offer salads, but many do not have healthy dressing options, and most salads have cheese. Many of these restaurants offer reasonably healthy breakfast options if you go for the scrambled eggs with no sausage or potato patty. Definitely avoid the pancakes. These options will obviously change over time, but the menus are trending healthier *(App 11-15 Rec.)*. Kentucky Fried Chicken (KFC) has a grilled chicken option. You can get the grilled chicken in a bucket, as with the fried chicken, and get green beans with the meal. Pass on the sweet kernel corn as this is inflammatory. Chick-Fil-A has a grilled chicken sandwich that is good if you avoid the dressing. If you are on the keto push, don't eat the bun. Boston Market has several healthy items to choose, from including turkey options, which are great if you pass on the gravy and mashed potatoes.

As you can see, there are many healthy anti-inflammatory options that you can pick up at fast food establishments. You may have to manipulate or special order some of the items, but this is much easier than cooking for yourself.

If you would like to order Chinese food, there is a wide range of options that have varying anti-inflammatory properties. Some good options include chicken with broccoli. You can have them add tofu that is not fried. Chicken with snow peas and shrimp with vegetables are also good options. Avoid some of the favorites such as fried rice, egg rolls, egg foo young, and noodle dishes such as chow mein or lo mein. Stick to dishes with steamed vegetables and meats such as chicken or shrimp. Duck is relatively high in fat and should be avoided unless you are just eating the duck breast with no skin. Avoid anything that is fried such as crab rangoon and General Tso's chicken. Sweet and sour chicken and pork are also fried and sugary and very inflammatory. Kung pao chicken is a reasonable option in most Chinese restaurants as it has mostly vegetables and some chicken. Ma-po tofu is a reasonable dish that has a bean-based sauce and chili peppers that are anti-inflammatory. Avoid orange beef as it is very sugary and heavy in saturated fats.

With Thai food you can find some healthy options such as chicken satay and tom yum soup. Pad Thai is loaded with carbohydrates due to the noodles, so you should avoid it. Many of the stir-fried dishes are fairly anti-inflammatory depending on the oil used to fry the meal. Most curry dishes are fairly good, but you must check on the additives such as oils or fatty meats. Most of the soups, such as curry-based soups, will tend to be relatively anti-inflammatory but will vary from restaurant to restaurant. You should try to avoid the fried spring rolls but the non-fried spring rolls are likely less inflammatory.

With Japanese food there are many healthy anti-inflammatory options that you can choose. You can go with nigari or sushi, which are the fish with the rice. The problem is the rice, which is inflammatory and should be avoided, particularly if you are on the keto push. Another option is to order primarily sashimi, which is just the fish with no rice. If it is an option, you can have brown or black rice with the fish instead of the white rice. Sushi in general is relatively healthy and primarily anti-inflammatory. It is a good idea to monitor your mercury intake if you eat a lot of sushi as the mercury can build up over the years and cause toxicity. Make sure you limit the amount of tuna or larger fish. In general, restaurants that serve multiple grades of tuna (super white tuna, fatty tuna, magaro, etc.) are more likely to have fish that has come from a larger tuna that will have higher mercury levels. If you go to a sushi restaurant that serves only magaro then the tuna source may be a smaller fish with less mercury If you want to keep mercury levels down, choose smaller fish such as salmon. You can also choose shrimp or eel. Other fish that may be high in mercury include; mackerel, big eye and bluefin tuna *(App 11-16 Ref.)*.

Most people order rolls or maki sushi when they go to a sushi restaurant. Maki sushi are rolls with multiple ingredients such as fish, fish eggs, avocado and cucumber. Many of these rolls have added mayonnaise or cream cheese. These are more of an American modification to cater to American tastes. Maki sushi can vary quite a bit from restaurant to restaurant. Some maki sushi can be very elaborate, featuring many types of fish such as tuna, yellowtail, salmon and crab. These rolls can be inflammatory based on what is in the roll. Any roll that is fried or contains fried foods is inflammatory. For example, a spider roll has fried soft shell crab and is inflammatory with saturated fats. A tempura roll or dynamite roll will likely have fried shrimp and is inflammatory. A Philadelphia roll has smoked salmon and cream cheese and is inflammatory. Rolls with non-fried foods and no dairy (cream cheese) or mayonnaise can be relatively non-inflammatory. Another option is temaki or a hand-roll, which is a cone of seaweed paper (nori) that is filled with rice and fish. You could order a spicy salmon hand roll with chili spicy sauce and avocado with brown or black rice if possible. The more elaborate a roll, the more likely it is inflammatory.

Other good options to eat at a Japanese restaurant include edamame, miso soup and seaweed salad. Miso soup has tremendous health benefits and consists of a thick paste made from soybeans that have been fermented with salt and a koji starter. Regular intake of miso has been shown to decrease the likelihood of lung, colon, liver and breast cancer.[167] Miso has probiotics that may help strengthen your gut flora, in turn boosting immunity and reducing the growth of harmful bacteria.[168] Seaweed salad (wakame) has many nutritional benefits including its high omega-3 fatty acids level, and many nutrients such as manganese, folate, magnesium, calcium, riboflavin and iron. This food supports the thyroid by providing iron and can reduce cholesterol and avoid heart disease. Wakame also contains polyphenols that exert similar anti-inflammatory and antioxidant benefits as green tea's catechin EGCG. Seaweed also contains a carotenoid called fucoxanthin that potentially reduces body fat and triglycerides and stimulates fat oxidation, especially dangerous visceral fat. It may also improve insulin resistance. Seaweed salad has tremendous anti-inflammatory benefits and is naturally tasty.

If you choose Japanese food, avoid the fried tempura or tonkatsu (deep fried pork cutlet) or noodle dishes. If you have a taste for ramen you can choose the soba noodle, which is the buckwheat flour that is higher in fiber, has more protein and is higher in minerals and vitamin B1 and B2. Soba also contains Rutin, which is very effective for anti-aging and lowering blood pressure. Broiled fish dishes are good choices such as broiled mackerel, which is high in omega-3 fatty acids. Tofu dishes are also very good and healthy. The teriyaki dishes are relatively healthy except that the teriyaki sauce will tend to have sugar in it. If the restaurant goes lighter with the teriyaki seasoning, then it will be better from an inflammatory point of view. Green tea is always good, but avoid the green tea ice cream as it obviously has sugar in it.

The Okinawa diet

Japanese women have an average lifespan of 86.8 years. The average life expectancy for women worldwide is 73.8 years. It is well known that the Japanese diet plays a huge role in this extended lifespan. A typical Japanese diet is low in saturated fat and high in nutrients that are antioxidant-rich. In Okinawa in the south of Japan there are more centenarians (living to over 100 years of age) than anywhere else in the world. The focus on the diet is on grains and vegetables (complex carbohydrates), soy products, followed by fish and meats *(App 11-16 Ref.)*. Milk and dairy products are at the bottom of the food pyramid. The Japanese have a low intake of saturated fats. In Japan, there is a culture of not overeating—you typically eat until you're 70 to 80% full. The intake of lots of fish and healthy vegetables are key to the Okinawa diet.[169] Try to incorporate as many aspects of this diet as you can into your own diet.[170]

One of the interesting features of the Okinawa diet is the prominence of sweet potatoes. The sweet potato has several features that are different from the typical Idaho potato. Sweet potatoes are root tubers that are part of the morning glory family and are only distantly related to the non-sweet potatoes. Other root tubers include beets, carrots and turnips. The potatoes used to make baked potatoes and French fries are from the nightshade family that include tomatoes and eggplant. Sweet potatoes are not the same as yams, which are cylindrical and are related to grasses and lilies. There are many different types of sweet potatoes, including Jewel, Garnet, Beauregard and Okinawan. The Okinawan sweet potatoes are purple with a high anthocyanin content, which gives the red, blue and violet colors. It is the anthocyanins that give the Okinawan sweet potato its potent antioxidant property that is comparable to blueberries. Sweet potatoes also contain cyanidin, which also reduces inflammation. In the Okinawa diet they get about 60% of their calories from sweet potatoes. Sweet potatoes have several other benefits, including being high in fiber, vitamin C, niacin (vitamin B3), vitamin B5, vitamin B6 and vitamin C as well as minerals such as magnesium, potassium, copper and manganese *(App 11-18 Ref.)*. The high fiber will help to lower LDL levels in the blood. One of the problems with potatoes is that they have a higher GI score, meaning that they are digested relatively quickly into sugars. Sweet potatoes are slightly lower on the GI score and slower to digest but are still not keto friendly. Sweet potatoes are also rich in vitamin A, which is important to support vision. To find Okinawan sweet potatoes you may need to make a trip to an oriental food market. Choose sweet potatoes that are firm with a uniform coloring and store them at room temperature.

Sweet potatoes can be prepared in many different ways. It is preferable to bake or grill them to a slightly crunchy texture with added salt, pepper and little garlic. This is a nice treat to eat with a turkey burger as a healthy replacement for French fries. Sweet potatoes can be prepared by boiling, steaming, mashing, or cooking in a wok for a stir-fry. You do not want to fry them as this can destroy their health benefits. To maximize the antioxidant effect of the sweet potatoes, you can leave the skin on as it contains a lot more antioxidants than the inside of the root. You can prepare a sweet potato similar to how you would eat a typical baked potato, split and baked with healthy ingredients such as garbanzo beans and spices topped with slices of avocado. You could split a sweet potato and add some grilled chicken strips with olive oil and garlic. You can also consider making a sweet potato soup with added veggies and garbanzo beans. There are many options for preparing sweet potatoes and many of these options are available online *(App 11-19 AIF.)*.

If you want to take out some healthy anti-inflammatory food options, you can order from one of Andrew Weil's restaurants called True Food Kitchen *(App 11-20 Rec.+)*. You could also use one of his cookbooks for options to create yourself *(App 11-21 Rec.+)*. You can try some of the recipes and experiment a bit with different approaches to meal preparation. If you start to cook anti-inflammatory meals on your own you will find it is very satisfying, and you are getting healthier at the same time.

12 DIFFERENT ANTI-INFLAMMATORY DIET PLANS BASED ON YOUR GOALS

Some people may need a more programmatic approach to instituting the anti-inflammatory diet into their daily plans. In this chapter, I have categorized four programs based on how quickly and how strictly you would like to adhere to the anti-inflammatory diet or whether you want the keto push. Each level has a different goal and can be fashioned to your level of commitment and your realistic expectations. Each level has suggested food items for a week and options for daily meals. In each level I will provide basic guidelines to keep you on track. Ideally, you will progress to higher levels as you become more committed to the anti-inflammatory diet.

LEVEL 1
Starter plan with low expectations

In this group, the meals are fashioned to allow you to break into the anti-inflammatory diet with a relatively smooth transition and with relative ease depending on where your initial baseline is situated. Many of the meals at this level are actually not anti-inflammatory but will introduce base foods that are anti-inflammatory. The base foods are "tricked up" to make them taste better. This will get you accustomed to eating these foods and then the "bad stuff" can be removed or replaced with more anti-inflammatory options as you progress to the later levels. If you have a terrible diet, then your initial transition will be more difficult no matter how you approach it.

Cut back on all simple carbohydrates limiting to one simple carb item per meal.

1. Limit to one dairy item per meal.
2. Limit to eating out three times a week.
3. Fast food option only once per week following the recommended guidelines.
4. Limit to one alcoholic beverage per day.
5. Limit to one sugary item per day.
6. Drink at least one glass of green tea a day.

DAY 1
BREAKFAST
You can choose from many healthier options with low to moderate inflammation: Greek yogurt with blueberries and multigrain toast with avocado spread. Coffee or green tea. Two glasses of water.
LUNCH
Turkey meat submarine sandwich with extra turkey, lettuce, olives, mustard, Italian dressing and one slice of cheese. Instead of regular potato chips add sweet potato chips or a handful of almonds.
SNACK
Pita chips with hummus.
DINNER
Grilled salmon served with grilled asparagus with mayonnaise-based dipping sauce *(App 12-1 AIF)*. Side of cauliflower pasta with pesto garlic sauce *(App 12-2 AIF+)*. Served with baby greens salad with balsamic vinegar and olive oil dressing. Have a glass of wine with dinner and a glass of water.
DESSERT
Low-fat almond butter ice cream *(App 12-3 AIF)*.

DAY 2
BREAKFAST
Cheese and mushroom omelet with multigrain toast and almond butter spread. Two glasses of water. Coffee or green tea.
LUNCH
Grilled chicken breast sandwich with lettuce and dressing. Sweet potato fries. Cup of matcha green tea. Two glasses of water with electrolyte supplement *(App 12-4 Rec. +)*.
SNACK
Crunchy chickpeas *(App 12-5 AIF +)*.
DINNER
Cauliflower crust pizza with low sugar or no sugar pizza sauce, chicken sausage, onions, mushrooms, red peppers, and low-fat Parmesan cheese *(App 12-6 AIF +)*. If you don't want to make your own crust, you can get a great cauliflower crust premade *(App 12-7 Rec. +)*. Served with baby greens salad and balsamic vinegar and olive oil dressing. Have a light beer with your meal and two glasses of water.
SNACK
Mixed berries with a sprinkle of cane sugar.

DAY 3

BREAKFAST

Steel cut oatmeal made with almond milk *(App 12-8 AIF)* covered with a teaspoon of maple syrup, dried raisins and cranberries. Multigrain toast with one egg over easy on top of it. Coffee or green tea.

LUNCH

Chicken tacos *(App 12-9 AIF)* with whole wheat tortillas (not fried) and tomato, onions, salsa and low-fat cheese option *(App 12-9 AIF)*. Served with a hearty chicken tortilla soup *(App 12-11 AIF+)*. If you would like a light lunch, just have the chicken tortilla soup with a glass of water.

SNACK

Protein bar *(App 12-12 Rec.)*.

DINNER

Grilled lean steak (tenderloin or sirloin) that is organic and grass-fed. Served with grilled sweet potato *(App 12-13 AIF)* and low-fat sour cream. Grilled kale chips with olive oil and salt. Have a glass of wine with dinner and a glass of water.

SNACK

One small piece of dark chocolate with cappuccino.

DAY 4

BREAKFAST

Scrambled eggs with ham and low-fat parmesan cheese. Multigrain toast with almond butter and banana slices *(App 12-14 AIF +)*. To keep the calories low, just have the almond butter banana toast without the eggs or vice versa. Coffee or green tea.

LUNCH

Hearty minestrone soup *(App 12-15 AIF +)* served with a side of sweet potato fries *(App 12-16 AIF)*. Serve with cup of green tea and electrolyte water *(App 12-17 Rec.)*.

SNACK

Handful of roasted almonds.

DINNER

Chinese food takeout order of beef and broccoli, egg foo young, spring rolls and egg drop soup *(App 12-18 Rec.+)*. You can order a fried rice dish, but do not combine with a noodle dish. Avoid the fried egg rolls. Order spring rolls instead. Serve with a cup of green tea and a glass of water.

SNACK

Green tea ice cream.

DAY 5
BREAKFAST
Scrambled egg/spinach sandwich on multigrain bread with low-fat parmesan cheese *(App 12-19 AIF)*. Coffee or matcha green tea.
LUNCH
Turkey sandwich wrap with tomato, onions and chickpea-based dressing *(App 12-20 AIF)*. Served with falafel. Have two glasses of water.
SNACK
Popcorn served with salt and olive oil sprinkle.
DINNER
Beef stew the vegetables cooked in a slow cooker *(App 12-21 AIF)*. Use organic beef and organic vegetables. Serve with keto dinner rolls *(App 12-22 AIF)*. Enjoy a glass of wine with your meal. Add a glass of water.
SNACK
Banana with almond butter

DAY 6
BREAKFAST
Egg bites *(App 12-23 AIF)* served with multigrain toast. Eggs bite options can be homemade or purchased from many different sources *(App 12-23 AIF)*. Coffee or green tea.
LUNCH
Sub sandwiches can be picked up, but take the wheat bread option and avoid processed meats such as pepperoni or salami. Avoid the chips. Two glasses of water.
SNACK
Handful of pistachios.
DINNER
Tandoori chicken *(App 12-24 AIF)* served with pilau rice *(App 12-25 AIF +)*. Also serve with grilled mixed vegetables. Baby green salad with cucumbers and chickpea dressing *(App 12-26 AIF)*. Have a glass of wine with dinner.
SNACK
Paleo lemon sorbet *(App 12-27 AIF)*.

DAY 7

BREAKFAST

Steel cut oatmeal with dried cranberries and sprinkle of brown sugar. Add small portion of Greek yogurt and multigrain toast. Coffee or matcha green tea. Glass of water as well.

LUNCH

Almond butter sandwich on multigrain bread and vegetable soup *(App 12-28 AIF)*. Two glasses of water with electrolytes.

SNACK

Cottage cheese and dried apricots.

DINNER

Pot roast *(App 12-29 AIF +)* with sweet potatoes *(App 12-30 AIF)*. Use a lean chuck roast with no bone. Serve with grilled broccoli with olive oil and salt. Serve with a baby lettuce salad and balsamic vinegar and olive oil dressing. Drink two glasses of water.

SNACK

Turkey jerky *(App 12-31 Rec.)* and cup of ginger peach turmeric tea *(App 12-32 Rec. +)*.

These meal options can be mixed and matched depending on your caloric needs. Some of the recommendations are for very active people who are working out every day. If you are more sedentary or are trying to lose weight, then your total caloric intake should be less. You may need to cut the snacks and decrease the amount of food eaten during each meal. You may consider skipping meals to decrease total caloric intake. It is helpful to try to decrease the amount of food eaten to decrease the size of your stomach. This will help you feel satisfied with less food intake. This first level is only the initial attempt at the anti-inflammatory diet. Your ultimate goal should be to move on the at least level 2 as staying at level 1 will not allow you to make the required progress necessary to become anti-inflamed.

LEVEL 2
Intermediate plan for the committed

At this level you are beyond committed and definitely see the benefits of incorporating the anti-inflammatory diet. You are not yet ready to go hard core but have enough enthusiasm to want to make a greater commitment to staying on the program. You still would like to cheat occasionally but want to be primarily uninflamed. This is where most of you will likely settle. Getting to level 3 and staying there is very difficult.

1. Only deviate from the diet twice a week.
2. Avoid most all sugars other than fresh fruits (blueberries, strawberries, etc.).
3. Cut out most white foods and replace with the healthier options such as multigrain bread, cauliflower crusts or chickpea pasta. Limit white rice and replace with couscous, black rice or brown rice.
4. Drink at least one glass of green tea a day and matcha at least three days a week.
5. Avoid most fried foods.
6. Eat mostly organic and avoid any corn-fed meats.

7. Avoid most desserts.
8. Alcohol twice a week with dinner.

DAY 1
BREAKFAST
Steel cut oatmeal made with almond milk with blueberries and strawberries. Have matcha green tea and two glasses of water.
LUNCH
Baby lettuce salad with grilled chicken, onions, cucumbers, tomato and avocado with balsamic vinegar and olive oil dressing. Cup of green tea and two glasses of water.
SNACK
Baby carrots with hummus and glass of water.
DINNER
Chicken fajitas *(App 12-33 AIF +)* with onions and red peppers on whole wheat tortillas. Use free-range organic chicken. Add salsa as needed. Add cheese substitute if desired. Serve with grilled mixed vegetables with balsamic vinegar. Serve with two glasses of water with electrolytes.
SNACK
Fuji apple with almond butter. Serve with cup of chamomile tea.

DAY 2

BREAKFAST

Omelet with spinach and mushrooms with no cheese. Served with toasted Ezekiel bread and natural berry spread with no added sugar *(App 12-34 Rec)*. Serve with cup of matcha green tea and two glasses of water.

LUNCH

Ginger chicken vegetable soup *(App 12-35 AIF +)* with almond butter on toasted Ezekiel bread. Cup of green tea. Add a glass of water with electrolytes.

SNACK

Boiled edamame *(App 12-36 AIF +)* with sesame oil and salt. Glass of water.

DINNER

Cedar plank salmon *(App 12-37 AIF +)* with brown sugar and Dijon mustard. Serve with grilled asparagus with extra-virgin olive oil, garlic and salt. Have a glass of wine with dinner. Add two glasses of water.

SNACK

Trail mix *(App 12-38 AIF)*. Serve with cup of white tea.

DAY 3

BREAKFAST

Shake with almond milk, one scoop ground flax seed, one tablespoon of olive oil, one teaspoon of chia seeds, frozen blueberries and strawberries and half of a banana. Eat with a slice of toasted Ezekiel bread. Serve with coffee or green tea and one glass of water.

LUNCH

Salad with baby lettuces, cucumber, onions, tomatoes and topped with a small piece of grilled salmon. Use a lemon vinaigrette dressing *(App 12-39 AIF +)*. Add a couple of walnuts on top of the salad. Drink a cup of matcha green tea and two cups of water.

DINNER

Turkey meatloaf with steamed artichokes and lemon, olive oil with garlic, salt and parsley dipping sauce *(App 12-40 AIF +)*. Lean ground turkey is used to make the meatloaf *(App 12-41 AIF +)*. Have a baby spinach salad with balsamic vinegar and olive oil dressing. Have two glasses of water with the meal.

SNACK

Kiwi fruit with a cup of ginger tea.

DAY 4
BREAKFAST
Hard-boiled eggs with a slice of avocado toast on Ezekiel bread. Glass of almond milk. Coffee or matcha green tea. Glass of water as well.
LUNCH
Sub sandwich with sliced turkey, lettuce, olives, tomato, avocado spread and Italian dressing. No cheese. Have with 10 roasted almonds. Two cups of water and a cup of green tea.
SNACK
Fruit and nut bar *(App 12-42 Rec. +)*. Glass of water.
DINNER
Stuffed chicken breasts premade or homemade. You can also make quinoa stuffed chicken breasts from scratch *(App 12-43 AIF +)*. Served with roasted French green beans with olive oil, garlic and salt. Baby lettuce salad with balsamic vinegar and olive oil dressing. Glass of red wine and two glasses of water with dinner.
SNACK
Mixed fruit bowl with strawberries, blueberries and kiwi. Cup of decaffeinated green tea.

DAY 5	
BREAKFAST	
Two eggs over easy with chicken sausage and toasted Ezekiel bread with natural, sugar-free strawberry jam *(App 12-44 AIF)*. Have a cup of matcha green tea and a glass of water.	
LUNCH	
Vegan egg salad sandwich with tofu, olive oil, turmeric and Dijon mustard *(App 12-45 AIF +)*. Have with kale chips and hummus. Two glasses of water with your meal.	
SNACK	
Low sugar energy bar *(App 12-46 Rec. +)*. Serve with glass of water.	
DINNER	
Turkey meatballs *(App 12-47 AIF +)* for pasta dish. Serve over chickpea pasta and pesto spinach sauce with olive oil and no tomato base *(App 12-48 AIF +)*. Serve with gluten-free garlic breadsticks *(App 12-49 AIF)*. Two glasses of water with electrolyte replacement.	
SNACK	
One piece of dark chocolate. Serve with cup of chamomile tea.	

DAY 6
BREAKFAST
Avocado and poached egg on Ezekiel toast *(App 12-50 AIF +)*. Serve with a sliced orange and coffee. Matcha green tea as well. One glass of water after the meal.
LUNCH
Apple turkey burger *(App 12-51 AIF +)* on whole wheat bun with avocado spread and lettuce and pickle. Serve with sweet potato fries *(App 12-52 AIF +)* and a glass of pomegranate juice and two glasses of water.
SNACK
Dried organic mango strips *(App 12-53 Rec.)*. Serve with glass of water.
DINNER
Tofu stir-fry with extra firm tofu and mixed vegetables served on brown rice of cauliflower rice *(App 12-54 AIF +)*. You could also use quinoa instead of rice. This should be cooked in a hot wok. You can serve with an Asian chopped salad *(App 12-55 AIF)*. Enjoy a glass of sake with your meal. Also two glasses of water.
SNACK
Edamame with sesame oil and salt. Cup of ginger tea.

DAY 7
BREAKFAST
Anti-inflammatory smoothie with hemp protein, leafy greens, frozen berries and ginger *(App 12-56 AIF)*. Serve with two hard-boiled eggs and coffee. You can have smoked salmon instead of the hard-boiled eggs if you wish. Have a matcha green tea to top off the meal and a tall glass of water as well.
LUNCH
Fresh beet salad with arugula and balsamic vinaigrette dressing *(App 12-57 AIF +)*. This salad can be served with tofu, chicken or grilled salmon. Have two glasses of water with electrolytes.
SNACK
Pomegranate bar *(App 12-58 Rec)*. Serve with glass of water.
DINNER
Dine out to a restaurant to have Mediterranean food. The meal consists of tabouli, hummus plate, baba ganoush, Greek salad and lemon chicken. If you wish to cook Mediterranean at home, you can make either a Greek shrimp farro bowl *(App 12-59 AIF +)* or one-pan Mediterranean cod *(App 12-60 AIF +)*. These are outstanding dishes that are moderately anti-inflammatory. Top the meal off with a Greek martini *(App 12-61 AIF)*. Drink two glasses of water with the meal.
SNACK
Italian apple olive oil cake *(App 12-62 AIF)*. Cup of peach turmeric tea.

At level 2 you are doing great. You may decide to settle at this stage. If you remain at this stage you will be much improved but still slightly inflamed. You will have many good days and some days where you experience some stuffiness in your nose and discomfort in your joints. Your will gain some benefit in your protection from a bad outcome with Covid-19 as you will be less inflamed. To progress to a state of minimal inflammation you will need to go to level 3.

LEVEL 3
Hard core who do not bend the rules

At this level you are totally committed to sticking to this diet and will likely gain tremendous benefit in a very short period of time. This diet plan can be somewhat monotonous due to the more restricted options. You can mix it up, but stay with the least inflammatory options. You can change up some of the recipes in levels 1 and 2 to be less inflammatory by eliminating some of the inflammatory ingredients such as sugar, tomato-based additives or simple carbohydrates. In this level you will find yourself repeating many meal options on a weekly basis. You will be able to identify your favorites and learn to shop efficiently. Cooking your own meals will be more common with this level as you will need to more precisely control the ingredients in your foods. For example, you will be avoiding all corn-fed chicken and farm-raised fish. This may prove to be one of the most difficult tasks at this level of the anti-inflammatory diet. You are eating to live "longer" and not living to eat. If you progress to level 3, you are set up to lose any existing comorbidities and avoid any new ones from popping up. You can potentially prolong your life as well.

1. No simple carbohydrates (sugars, pasta, rice or bread) and primarily complex carbohydrates such as broccoli, kale, spinach, cauliflower, artichoke, green beans and asparagus.
2. No red meats or chicken skin.
3. No desserts. Apples and blueberries are acceptable.
4. All organic foods.
5. No corn-fed chicken or fish.
6. At least two glasses of green tea or matcha per day.
7. Limit eating out to once a week.
8. One alcoholic beverage per week.
9. Deviate from the diet only once a week. Deviations from the

diet are minor infractions such as some rice with your sushi or some raisins with your steel cut oatmeal.

DAY 1
BREAKFAST
Green tea shake with 200 ml to 500 ml of green tea depending on how many glasses of shake you would like to have. If you would like to drink two large glasses of the shake, use about 500 ml or 16 ounces of decaffeinated green tea. Add one large scoop of egg white protein, one large scoop of ground flax seed, and one tablespoon of chia seeds. Then add one to two cups of frozen blueberries. To add more calories you can add avocado or olive oil. Blend it to a nice consistency using a blender. The shake will hold you over until lunch. Follow this up with at least two large glasses of water. Add a cup of matcha green tea instead of coffee.
LUNCH
Baby lettuce salad with chicken breast (pieces) and balsamic vinegar and olive oil dressing. You can add slices of avocado to increase the calories and good fat content. Drink at least two large glasses of water.
SNACK
Ten roasted almonds or an apple. One large glass of water with electrolyte supplement.
DINNER
Wild caught fresh salmon grilled with olive oil, salt and pepper. You will need fresh salmon to appreciate the taste of the meat with such few spices added. Large portion of grilled broccoli sprinkled with olive oil and salt. One large glass of water.
SNACK
One Fuji apple. Serve with cup of chamomile tea.

DAY 2
BREAKFAST:
Green tea shake with decaffeinated green tea and blueberries. Add one large scoop of egg white protein, one large scoop of ground flax seed, and one tablespoon of chia seeds. To add more calories you can add avocado or olive oil. Follow up with at least two large glasses of water. Add a cup of matcha green tea instead of coffee.
LUNCH:
Baby lettuce salad with chicken breast (pieces) and balsamic vinegar and olive oil dressing. At least one large glass of water.
SNACK:
Six walnuts and cup of black tea and glass of water.
DINNER:
Grilled chicken breasts prepared with olive oil, garlic, salt and Greek seasoning *(App 12-63 Rec. +)*. Grilled cauliflower with Garbanzo beans sprinkled with olive oil, turmeric and salt. Baby greens salad with olive oil and vinegar dressing and two slices of avocado. Two glasses of water.
SNACK:
Granny smith apple served with cup of ginger tea.

DAY 3

BREAKFAST:

Two eggs over easy with chicken sausage. Followed up with at least two large glasses of water. Add a cup of matcha green tea instead of coffee.

LUNCH:

Baby lettuce salad with grilled salmon and lemon vinaigrette dressing *(App 12-64 AIF +)*. Two slices of avocado to top the salad. At least one large glass of water.

DINNER:

Turmeric roasted turkey breast with olive oil, garlic, salt and pepper *(App 12-65 AIF +)*. Boiled artichokes with olive oil, crushed garlic, salt and parsley dipping sauce or grilled artichoke option *(App 12-66 AIF +)*. Baby greens salad with olive oil and balsamic vinegar dressing. Two glasses of water with the meal.

SNACK:

Cup of blueberries and cup of ginger tea.

DAY 4

BREAKFAST

Smoked salmon on a slice of toasted Ezekiel bread. Follow with at least two large glasses of water. Add a cup of matcha green tea instead of coffee.

LUNCH

Baby lettuce salad with low mercury tuna *(App 12-67 Rec. +)* or sardines and lemon vinaigrette dressing. Two slices of avocado to top the salad. At least two large glasses of water.

DINNER

Cauliflower crust pizza with olive oil, garlic, salt, pepper and oregano instead of tomato-based pizza sauce *(App 12-68 AIF)*. Chicken pieces, onions, red peppers and mushrooms. Bake the crust on both sides for 10 minutes or until brown before adding sauce. Then place the sauce and add the other ingredients. The chicken is precooked prior to placing on the pizza. You can add soy cheese if you wish. Served with baked kale chips sprinkled with olive oil and salt. Two glasses of water with electrolytes.

SNACK

Fuji apple. Cup of peach ginger turmeric tea *(App 12-69 Rec.)*.

DAY 5

BREAKFAST

Two hard-boiled eggs served with slice of toasted Ezekiel bread with cilantro lime avocado spread *(App 12-70 AIF +)*. Add a cup of matcha green tea and glass of water.

LUNCH

Almond butter sandwich on toasted Ezekiel bread. Cup of green tea and glass of water with electrolytes *(App 12-71 Rec)*.

SNACK

Petite carrots with hummus and cup of matcha green tea. Glass of water as well.

DINNER

Grilled turkey burgers *(App 12-72 AIF +)* on whole wheat bun with grilled onions and mustard. Serve with grilled asparagus with olive oil and salt. Baby greens salad with balsamic vinegar and olive oil dressing and some walnuts.

SNACK

Cup of fresh blueberries. Cup of ginger tea.

DAY 6
BREAKFAST
Steel cut oatmeal prepared al dente with walnuts and blueberries. Served with a matcha tea with almond milk. Glass of water as well.
LUNCH
Smashed avocado chickpea salad sandwich with cranberries and lemon on whole grain bread *(App 12-73 AIF +)*.
Or have the green tea shake with one large scoop of egg white protein, one large scoop of ground flax seed, and one tablespoon of chia seeds and frozen blueberries. For more calories you can add avocado or olive oil. The shake will hold you over until dinner. The green tea shake for lunch is a great option during the summer months when you would like to eat a light lunch so you do not get sluggish. It is also quick to make and drink.
SNACK
Celery sticks with walnut butter. Cup of matcha green tea. Glass of water as well.
DINNER
Sushi dinner ordered from Japanese restaurant. Miso soup and seaweed salad. Edamame with salt. Six pieces of salmon sashimi, two pieces of mackerel sashimi, two spicy salmon hand rolls (chili spicy, not mayo spicy) with avocado and black rice. If you order other fish keep in mind that larger fish (tuna, yellowtail) have higher mercury levels. If you choose rolls (maki sushi), try to avoid the options with cream cheese or fried ingredients.
SNACK
Cup of strawberries. Glass of water with electrolytes *(App 12-74 Rec.)*.

CHAPTER 12: Different Anti-inflammatory Diet Plans Based on Your Goals 151

DAY 7
BREAKFAST
Egg white omelet with spinach, mushrooms and onions. No cheese. Avocado toast made with toasted Ezekiel bread. Matcha green tea and a glass of water.
LUNCH
Buddha bowl with kale, avocado, orange and wild rice *(App 12-75 AIF +)*. Other anti-inflammatory lunch options can be found as well *(App 12-76 AIF)*. Have two glasses of water.
SNACK
Handful of roasted chickpeas *(App 12-77 AIF)*. Glass of water.
DINNER
Two spatchcocked wild organic chickens prepared with lemon slices under the skin, covered with olive oil and thyme. The leftovers are used as protein for lunch salads throughout the week. Grilled French green beans with olive oil, salt and garlic. Baby lettuce salad with olive oil and vinegar dressing. Two glasses of water.
SNACK
Cup of blueberries. Cup of chamomile tea.

As one can see, the level 3 meals are more boring and monotonous. Once you reach level 3 you will know what meals work best for lowering your body's inflammation. The key is to have two to three options for every meal every day to keep some variety. For example, during the summer months when it is hot, having a green tea blueberry shake will cool you off. Some days you may want to pass on a meal. This is OK to do if you have a good snack. For example, on some days you can eat a handful of roasted almonds for lunch. This gives you some calories to hold you over to dinner. Breakfast is a very important meal, so do not pass on it if you plan on having a snack for lunch. You will need calories and protein for breakfast. If you need breakfast on the run, keep hard-boiled eggs or smoked salmon available. You can take the hard-boiled eggs and eat them on the road. You can cook them and peel the shells and store them in the refrigerator in a plastic bag. You can also toast a piece of Ezekiel bread and put either smoked salmon or almond butter on it. You can also take an almond butter sandwich for lunch if you are in a hurry. You can use your leftovers as a meal during the week if you are in a hurry or just do not want to cook.

Practicing the anti-inflammatory diet at level 3 requires a great deal of self-control and discipline. Not many people can get to this level and stay on it. What will tend to happen is that you will get to level 3 and then drop back to level 2 for periods of time. This is OK as long as you do not completely fall off the wagon. The difficult times are when you go out to eat or are invited to a party or dinner at someone else's home. Then there is great pressure to eat what is available at the event. If you are attending a wedding or reception, you can call ahead to see what is being served. You can then get an idea if there are any anti-inflammatory options available. To avoid the worse scenario you can eat before you go or bring some almonds with you. Staying at level 3 is difficult and will challenge you at times. However, if you are able to stay on the plan you will surely make significant strides forward.

LEVEL 4
Anti-inflammatory diet with keto push (AI-keto)

At this level you will progress to the anti-inflammatory diet with the keto push to essentially cut most all carbs except complex carbohydrates (vegetables). This will help send you into a state of ketosis and start to burn fat instead of glucose. The difference between this diet and the conventional keto diet is that the foods eaten are anti-inflammatory. You will be counting net carbs and you should try to stay below 50 net carbs per day. This can be difficult but is doable. By shifting to a state of ketosis, you will burn body fat and lose abdominal fat and trim your waistline. If your total caloric intake is less than the calories that you burn you will lose weight as well. A good option is to pass on a meal several times a week. For example, on a weekend you could have a hearty late breakfast then fast through to dinner. This will allow you to stay under the 50 net carbs for the day and also lower your total caloric intake. This is something to consider on days that you might be consuming more carbs than normal. Fasting is one of the most efficient ways to reach a ketotic state. If you are diabetic or have low blood sugar, you should avoid fasting as an option.

The anti-inflammatory diet with keto push has a different proportioning of food groups than the conventional keto diet. **In this plan you will try to have 60% good fats, 25% proteins and 15% carbohydrates.** This will require that you add extra-virgin olive oil, avocado and lots of foods rich in omega-3 fatty acids to your diet plan. All of the vegetables will be sprinkled with extra-virgin olive oil. You can add slices of avocado to many of the meals. Make sure you are taking the omega-3 fatty acid supplement capsules as well. The addition of balsamic vinegar will be important to minimize digestion of some of the complex carbohydrates that you will be consuming.

You can measure your progress by testing your urine using test strips *(App 12-78 Rec.)*. It is a good idea to measure your blood ketone levels at least once a week *(App 12-79 Rec.)*. You can use an easy-to-use ketone blood test device to accomplish this *(App 12-80 Rec. +)*. By measuring your urine and blood ketone levels you will be able to insure that you are in the nutritional ketone state.

Many of the meal plans listed below are linked to websites that feature keto-friendly diets. These sites are very helpful when looking for great recipes to plan your anti-inflammatory keto push meals. Some of most helpful sites are featured in this section *(App 12-81 AIF +)*. Some of the meals are cooked in an "Instant pot" but can also be prepared in another type of pressure cooker *(App 12-82 Rec.)*. The recommendations below do not set specific net carb totals. You will have to vary the meal choices and amounts of each food item to stay with the net carb requirements.

No simple carbohydrates (sugars, pasta, rice or bread) and primarily complex carbohydrates such as broccoli, kale, spinach, cauliflower, artichoke, green beans and asparagus are on the keto push. Add olive oil to the vegetables to increase fat intake.

1. Use grain replacements such as almond flour and other fibers like flax and chia seeds.
2. Incorporate avocado into at least two meals a day.
3. Get your fats from meats and olive oil. Add olive oil to most of your meals.
4. Limit red meats or chicken skin. No more than one meal a week with red meat.
5. No desserts. If you choose to eat an apple or blueberries you will have to cut net carbs somewhere else during the day. Eat a half apple or half cup of blueberries.
6. All organic foods.
7. No fruit juices or sugary drinks.
8. No corn-fed meats.
9. At least two glasses of green tea or matcha per day.
10. Limit to eating out to once a week.
11. Exercise regularly focusing on core exercises (plank, etc.).
12. Add two omega-3 fatty acid capsules per day
13. Limit total carb intake to less than 50 grams per day. You can go over 50 grams but below 60 grams twice a week separated by at least two days.

14. Consider periodic fasting to lower caloric intake and decrease carbohydrate intake. Passing on lunch three times a week is a good option. You can also pass on the snacks throughout the week to decrease caloric intake and carb intake.

DAY 1
BREAKFAST
Fried egg with avocado on a toasted slice of Breadlam cube bread *(App 12-83 Rec)*. Served with a cup of matcha green tea. Coffee with no sugar or cream. Glass of water as well.
LUNCH
Baby lettuce salad with three ounces of grilled chicken breast and avocado with balsamic vinegar and olive oil dressing. You can substitute an apple cider vinegar dressing for the salad *(App 12-84 AIP)*. Serve with two glasses of water.
SNACK
One boiled egg or a scoop of no nightshade guacamole *(App 12-85 AIP +)*. Cup of green tea and glass of water.
DINNER
Chicken breasts grilled with olive oil and Greek seasoning served with grilled broccoli with olive oil and salt. Baby kale salad with avocado and pine nuts. Or chose grilled Chardonnay chicken *(App 12-86 AIP +)*. Water with electrolyte supplement.
SNACK
Six almonds (six grams of net carbs). Glass of water.

DAY 2
BREAKFAST
Anti-inflammatory low-carb keto-friendly porridge with six grams of net carbs *(App 12-88 AIP)*. Served with a cup of matcha green tea and glass of water.
LUNCH
Superfood kale salad with avocado and lemon juice *(App 12-89 AIP +)*. Served with a cup of green tea and glass of water. Consider fasting through lunch as an alternative.
SNACK
Keto friendly almond butter ball *(App 12-90 AIP)*. Net carbs are 2.5 grams. Glass of water.
DINNER
Instant pot salmon with chili-lime sauce *(App 12-91 AIP +)*. Served with crispy turmeric cauliflower *(App 12-92 AIP +)* with no nightshade guacamole *(App 12-93 AIP +)*. Have a glass of sparkling water as well.
SNACK
Slice of avocado on a celery stick. Glass of water. Cup of chamomile tea before bed.

DAY 3

BREAKFAST

Green tea shake with egg white protein, ground flaxseed, chia seeds, avocado and half cup of frozen blueberries. Serve with cup of green tea and glass of water.

LUNCH

Smoked salmon and avocado slices on a toasted slice of Breadllam cube bread *(App 12-94 AIP)*. You can sprinkle some chopped hard-boiled eggs on top. Serve with cup of matcha green tea and a glass of water.

SNACK

Veggie sticks with low-carb no nightshade guacamole *(App 12-95 AIP)*. Glass of water.

DINNER

Lemon sheet pan chicken with broccoli *(App 12-96 AIP)*. Romaine salad with balsamic vinegar and extra virgin olive oil dressing with avocado slices. Served with sparkling water, green tea and a glass of water.

SNACK

Half cup of raspberries. Glass of water. Cup of ginger tea before bed.

DAY 4	
BREAKFAST	
Two egg omelet with green peppers, mushrooms and dairy-free keto-friendly cheese *(App 12-97 AIP)*. Served with a cup of matcha green tea and glass of water.	
LUNCH	
Keto sushi rolls with sushi grade salmon, nori seaweed, cucumber, avocado, romaine lettuce and no rice. Served with a bowl of low-carb miso soup *(App 12-98 AIP)*. Two glasses of water.	
DINNER	
Instant pot Greek chicken *(App 12-99 AIP +)*. Serve with balsamic roasted cabbage steaks *(App 12-100 AIP +)*. Serve with a baby lettuce salad, avocado and lemon vinaigrette dressing *(App 12-101 AIP +)*. Also have two glasses of water with electrolytes *(App 12-102 Rec)*.	
SNACK	
Kale chips prepared with olive oil and salt *(App 12-103 AIF +)*. You can also purchase premade kale chips *(App 12-104 AIF Rec.)*. Glass of water.	

DAY 5
BREAKFAST
Low-carb keto overnight oatmeal *(App 12-105 AIF)* with soy milk. You can add some blueberries and blackberries. Matcha green tea and glass of water.
LUNCH
Keto chicken soup *(App 12-106 AIF +)*. Served with cauliflower breadsticks *(App 12-107 AIF)* and no nightshade guacamole *(App 12-108 AIF)*. Two glasses of water. Consider fasting through lunch as an alternative.
SNACK
Hard-boiled egg with a cup of matcha green tea with almond milk or flax milk *(App 12-109 Rec.)*.
DINNER
Beef bourguignon stew *(App 12-110 AIF)* served with cauliflower rice. Serve with grilled asparagus. Baby greens salad with avocado and Italian dressing *(App 12-111 AIF)*. Glass of water as well.
SNACK
Slice of honeydew. Cup of turmeric tea and glass of water.

DAY 6
BREAKFAST
Smoked salmon scrambled eggs *(App 12-112 AIF)*. Served with a slice of toasted Breadlam cube bread and two avocado slices. Have a cup of matcha green tea and water.
LUNCH
Sheet pan taco bowl with chicken strips *(App 12-113 AIF +)* and cauliflower rice. Avocado slices on top of taco bowl. Serve with a cup of green tea and glass of electrolyte water *(App 12-114 Rec.)*.
SNACK
Keto nut butter snack *(App 12-115 Rec. +)*. Cup of green tea. Glass of water as well.
DINNER
Herbed organic chicken and mushrooms *(App 12-116 AIF +)*. Serve with steamed artichoke (three grams net carbs) with olive oil, garlic and salt dipping sauce. Baby lettuce green salad with avocado and apple cider vinegar salad dressing *(App 12-117 AIF)*. Have two glasses of water with the meal.
SNACK
A small portion of 10 green olives (1.1 grams net carbs). Glass of water.

DAY 7

BREAKFAST

Keto-friendly egg bites *(App 12-118 AIF)* with egg whites and chia seeds. Serve with a cup of matcha green tea and a glass of water.

LUNCH

Dairy free avocado chicken salad *(App 12-119 AIF Video +)* served on lettuce. Serve with a cup of green tea and glass of water. Consider fasting through lunch as an alternative.

SNACK

Green tea matcha meringues *(App 12-120 AIF)*. Serve with two glasses of water. One glass with electrolytes.

DINNER

Turmeric spiced Mahi-Mahi *(App 12-121 AIF +)*. Serve with grilled French green beans *(App 12-122 AIF +)*. Purple romaine with avocado and balsamic vinegar and olive oil dressing. Two glasses of water.

SNACK

Low-carb crackers *(App 12-123 AIF)* with no nightshade guacamole *(App 12-124 AIF)*. Six crackers have just over three grams of net carbs. Have a glass of water as well.

The anti-inflammatory diet with keto push (AI-keto diet) is challenging due to the limitation of 50 net carbs per day. On days that you can anticipate eating more carbs than prescribed, you should consider passing on a meal such as lunch. Fasting is an effective way to get into a ketotic state. You will occasionally find yourself going over the 50 net carb limit. This is OK as long as you are staying anti-inflamed. Remember, the key is to stick with anti-inflammatory foods that just happen to get you to a state of ketosis and keep you there.

Finding your level when it comes to this diet can be tricky. Many of you will fluctuate from level to level. If you have an important event coming up such as a wedding, reunion or athletic competition, you can go to level 3 or 4 for the month leading up to it. This will set you up to feel and look your best during the event. If you would like to improve some of your comorbidities and improve your chances of defeating Covid-19, then you should try to move yourself from level 1 to at least level 2. This will give you a good opportunity to defeat the SARS-CoV-2 virus.

Note: these recommendations are meant to provide the dieter with guidelines to design daily meal plans. You can mix and match meal options based on how your day is set up. You can shift to different levels based on the time of year, your long-term plans and social circumstances. **Remember to consult with your physician prior to undertaking any of these dietary recommendations.** Good luck and stay uninflamed.

13 INFLAMMATION AND COVID-19

The Covid-19 pandemic has affected the lives of the entire world's population like never before. Studies have shown that those who are at greatest risk for a more complicated course with the Covid-19 infection are those who are obese with comorbidities, such as hypertension, diabetes and lung diseases such as asthma and other inflammatory disorders *(App 13-1 Ref.)*. A study based on 5,700 Covid-19 patients hospitalized in the New York City area showed that the majority of them had more than one comorbidity.[171] Researchers looked at the electronic health records (EMR) of 5,700 patients who were hospitalized with the SARS-CoV-2 virus with the Northwell health system in March and early April of 2020. The median age of the patients was 63, and 94% of the patients had at least one other comorbidity. The most common comorbidities were hypertension (53%), obesity (42%), diabetes (32%), morbid obesity (19%), and coronary artery disease (10.4%). The outcomes for patients that were placed on ventilators were very bad with a death rate of 88%. In the group of patients under the age of 20 there were no deaths. Morbidity was much higher in those over 60 years of age.

In August of 2020, the CDC released data stating that only 6% of COVID-19 deaths were caused by the virus, and the other 94% had other contributing factors (comorbidities) that lead to death.[172] This means that only 6% of the cases of COVID-19 that died did not have any other reported comorbidities. The actual mortality rates for Covid-19 are fluid and change as more people are tested and the virus mutates. Many epidemiologists have tried to determine the infection fatality rate (IFR). In a review of twenty-three studies with seroprevalence data, IFR ranged from 0.02% to 0.86% (median 0.26%).[173] In patients less than 70 years old the IFR ranged from 0.00-0.23% with median of 0.04%. The median fatality rate was 0.26% *(App 13-2 Ref.)*. The impact of comorbidities on the outcomes of patients who contracted Covid-19 was dramatic. People with normal weight and no comorbidities tended to do well with few symptoms and no prolonged complications. It is clear that one of the best ways to protect ourselves from having a bad outcome with the Covid-19 infection is to lessen the severity of or eliminate comorbidities. There is also some evidence that there may be a link to inflammation and how those who are inflamed may be more prone to a complicated course of this disease *(App 13-3 Ref.)*.

Inflammaging

There has been a steady increase in the incidence of age-related chronic inflammatory diseases such as diabetes, heart and lung disease, arthritis, osteoporosis, dementia and cancer. These increases have been ascribed to different genetic and environmental factors (diet, pollution, stress, etc.) that are closely linked to socioeconomic factors. **Chronic inflammation over many years in combination with the aging of our immune systems result in premature aging and is defined as "inflammaging."**[174] (Figure 17) Inflammaging is associated with frailty, morbidity, and mortality in elderly subjects. Factors that influence inflammaging include; how much visceral fat we have, the functioning status of our mitochondria that act as our chemical power plants, and the status of our gut wall bacteria *(App 13-4 Ref. Video +)*. Visceral fat forms when we eat a large quantity of inflammatory foods over a period of time. The visceral fat secretes many harmful substances that can damage the cells in our body. If our mitochondria are damaged then we may see more severe levels of dysfunction in our organs. Our gut walls have bacteria that help with digestion. These bacteria are in a layer of mucous along the walls of our gut. If this mucous layer thins out, the bacteria can invade the walls of our bowels and cause an abnormal immune response and trigger increased inflammation. All of these factors can contribute to **immunosenesence and inflammaging**.

Methods of mitigating chronic inflammation include; exercise, sleep, diet and fasting. Exercise helps to decrease the visceral fat and decrease stress. Sleep helps to decrease stress and improve overall cellular function. Diet and exercise are the primary means to decrease visceral fat and decrease inflammation. Our diet is believed to have a major influence on both the development and prevention of age-related chronic inflammatory diseases.[175] Inflammatory foods increase oxidative stress and inflammatory signaling. Dietary interventions such as the anti-inflammatory diet can mitigate the inflammaging phenotype and may protect us from many age-related diseases. Aging is complex and multifactorial. It is clear that one of the best ways to slow down the aging process and development of age-related chronic inflammatory diseases is through the anti-inflammatory diet.[176]

There is an association between inflammaging and the increased susceptibility of older men to Covid-19.[177] The ACE2 receptor that the SARS-CoV-2 virus attaches to and infects cells is expressed much more highly in men than women. Severe acute respiratory syndrome after SARS-CoV-2 infection is accompanied by a high mortality in elderly men with age-related comorbidities. In many of these patients, uncontrolled hyperinflammation induces severe or lethal outcomes. The aging process leads to the gradual development of a chronic subclinical systemic inflammation (inflammaging) and deterioration of the immune system (immune senescence). These appear to be significant factors in the suboptimal outcomes in the older men with Covid-19. It is particularly important in this population to take steps to avoid lethal outcomes if the SARS-CoV-2 virus comes back in the future. These efforts can be initiated through the institution of the anti-inflammatory diet as well as other lifestyle changes.

We all know of many older people who are active and full of life yet may have one or two comorbidities. Many of these individuals may be terrified of the SARS-CoV-2 virus and are looking for ways to protect themselves from the next pandemic. Obviously, wearing a mask and social distancing will be important measures to limit exposure to the virus. The next step to protect yourself will be through strengthening your immune system (avoiding immune senescence) and minimizing and preventing comorbidities (inflammaging). **Behind the mask, the anti-inflammatory diet can act as your second line barrier to protect you from contracting the virus** (Figure 18). If you are infected, you will have a better chance of fighting off the virus. Even if the SARS-CoV-2 virus never returns, you will be much healthier and less inflamed. You may even live longer and help to protect future generations from inflammation and disease.

Epigenetics

Even if you have a genetic tendency toward developing comorbidities such as hypertension, diabetes and stroke, the anti-inflammatory diet and exercise may allow you to overcome these genetic tendencies. Some people feel that they are doomed because of their genes, so why make the effort? This mentality is engrained in many generations of families that tend to have shorter lifespans. You are not doomed and you may be able to overcome these tendencies *(App 13-5 Ref. +)*. There is actual evidence that you can change your genes by changing your diet. This area of study is called epigenetics *(App 13-6 Ref. +)*.[178]

Epigenetics is the term used to describe inheritance by mechanisms other than through the DNA sequence of our genes and it works through chemical tags added to chromosomes that in effect switch genes on or off *(App 13-7 Ref. Video +)*. Some may think that your genes are the end all and be all of who you have become. Actually, you can do a lot to control how your genome expresses itself. If you have a genetic tendency to become diabetic, with diet control you may be able to avoid this genetic tendency from expressing itself. If you have a genetic tendency to develop hypertension and heart disease, you may be able to avoid these conditions as well. Even more significant may be the influence your behavior could have on your children and your children's children (Figure 19). **What you do to influence**

the expression of certain good or bad genes will potentially be passed on to future generations. It is apparent in some families that bad epigenetic information is being passed down to future generations. This may be occurring in your own gene pool. For example, your grandmother's dietary habits may have added type 2 diabetes into your genetic makeup that may now be affecting you *(App 13-7 Ref. +)*. Additionally, your bad diet may pass on type 2 diabetes to your children. Alternatively, you could turn off those genes by depressing certain chemical tags to stop the passage of this bad genetic tendency to future generations. If you could take a pill that would turn off the genes that would otherwise give your children diabetes, heart disease or asthma, you would surely take it. The anti-inflammatory diet could have a similar effect as that pill. This in itself is a good reason to get on the anti-inflammatory diet.

A good example of epigenetics is demonstrated in two identical twins. If the twins are brought up in completely different social environments, they will obviously be different. If one twin eats an anti-inflammatory diet and exercises daily and the other twin eats a high saturated fat diet and does not exercise, the one twin will likely be healthier with fewer comorbidities and the other may be obese with many comorbidities. These differences in their appearance and health status develop over their lives despite both having the exact same genes. This is epigenetics. Bottom line: You have control over your health status despite what you may think your genes doom you to become. Understanding this concept may be critical to overcome some of our preconceptions about our fate and could impact ones effort made to make significant changes in lifestyle and diet.

Are zinc and vitamin C effective in fighting Covid-19?

With other coronaviruses, zinc has proven to help slow the replication of the virus and potentially shorten the disease process.

There are many zinc-based products out there that have been shown to shorten the course of the common cold *(App 13-11 Ref.)*.[179] There is some evidence that zinc may help to prevent the progression of the SARS-CoV-2 virus *(App 13-12 Ref. +)*. It is more likely that zinc may be able to help prevent the SARS-CoV-2 virus from ever gaining traction if it gets into our bodies. Taking a couple of zinc lozenges with you when you fly or take a train is likely a good idea. You can carry some lozenges with you and if someone sneezes or coughs on you, simply pop a lozenge into your mouth to coat your throat with the zinc. You can use the low-sugar or sugar-free versions of the zinc lozenges to keep sugar levels down.

Vitamin C may also be beneficial in fighting viruses *(App 13-13 Ref.)*. The benefits of vitamin C have been discussed for many years and is known to be a potent antioxidant. People have been taking high doses of vitamin C to help fight off viruses and that is thought to help with SARS-CoV-2 as well. In some studies, patients with Covid-19 are being given high doses of vitamin C intravenously to try to shorten the course of the disease. Taking vitamin C supplements will not harm you so you can take 1000mg of a vitamin C supplement twice a day to help stave off disease. This applies to many diseases, including cancer, so as long as it will not hurt you it is worth taking. You can also eat a lot of oranges, grapefruit and kiwi as well as broccoli, cauliflower and kale. These food items are high in vitamin C and are generally anti-inflammatory as well as being high in fiber.

Pandemic stress can increase inflammation

Let's look back to the spring of 2020 during the Covid-19 pandemic. We were all told to shelter in place in our homes and apartments for the months of March, April and May. Some of us were fortunate enough to go back to near-normal in late May and June of 2020. For most in larger cities, the lockdown extended into June and July. Many were going stir-crazy and some were protesting to get back to work. Many had lost their jobs, with millions of Americans filing for unemployment benefits by the end of April, sending the totals above 30 million since the Covid-19 pandemic began to shutter businesses across the country in early March 2020. This was an unprecedented time and the economy continued to suffer, with our jobless rate pushing 22%—the highest since the great depression of the 1930s. We were trying to observe social distancing and were wearing masks when out in public. We could not go to restaurants and spent a lot of time waiting in our cars to get carryout orders. As restaurants opened we had to continue with social distancing, so capacity of 25% to 50% seating was typical. There were no sports. The entire NCAA tournament was cancelled as well as the 2020 summer Olympics in Tokyo. The Kentucky Derby was run with no spectators in the stands. The 2020 NFL draft was a virtual event. Broadway and the Las Vegas strip were shut down, as were all movie theaters. We all watched a lot of Netflix, Hulu and Amazon TV. All of our meetings were held via Zoom and no one was flying. It was not unusual to see one or two passengers on a regional flight in the U.S. Gyms and fitness centers were shut down. If you wanted to exercise, you needed to be creative, and just taking a walk was a difficult task as many parks and trails were closed. A new normal now existed. Most of us were just trying to stay safe and keep our families safe. We wanted to get back to work and make a living so we could support our families. These were tough times.

Given these conditions, it's easy to see why people were stressed. But the effects can be detrimental on a physical level as well as a psychological one. Increased stress has been linked to increased appetite and weight gain (Figure 20). When you are stressed, your body releases the stress hormone cortisol. When cortisol is released, it increases your appetite. You will tend to eat more sugar. Your visceral fat increases and you then form more cortisol and crave more sugar. This vicious cycle can perpetuate the weight gain and increase your body's inflammation as sugars are inflammatory. Included in the cravings for sugars are the cravings for carbohydrates. This also increases your body's inflammation. You must work hard to break this cycle by decreasing your body's cortisol levels by decreasing stress. This was difficult during the Covid-19 pandemic. In fact, nearly seven in 10 employees surveyed by mental health provider Ginger said that the Covid-19 pandemic has been the most stressful time of their entire professional career—even more stressful than 9/11 or the 2008 great recession.[180]. The increased stress associated with the Covid-19 pandemic also paralleled dramatic increases in prescriptions for antianxiety, antidepressants and sleeping aids. It is this highly stressful time that resulted in such high levels of individual stress that then triggered poor dietary habits and weight gain. Massive job loss and businesses shuttering created tremendous mental health issues and long-term effects that we can only now begin to determine. Was the cure worse than the disease? Only time will tell. In either case, it is apparent that the entire world has suffered.

The Covid-19 pandemic also affected the way we got our foods to the table in our homes. While we were in lockdown many people started to cook for themselves *(App 13-14 Ref. +)*. Many that rarely cooked in the past started to venture into cooking their own meals and developed new skills in the kitchen. This was a once-in-a-lifetime event that changed many things in our lives, including how we prepare our meals. Experimentation was very big, with many people learning to cook and bake. The Hunter food study report showed that during the pandemic, 54% of people were cooking more and 46% were baking more. (Figure 21) They showed that 50% were more confident in the kitchen and 51% stated that they would continue to cook more. This is not good for the restaurant industry, but is great if you want to take this opportunity to eat healthier. The study showed that 47% looked for ways to cook healthier. These are good changes that align directly with this opportunity to make a move to the anti-inflammatory diet. But while many were cooking more often, 40% of people were eating more indulgent foods that are not anti-inflammatory. This may in part be linked to the increased stress associated with the lockdown during the pandemic.

If we can get an effective vaccine, we should be safe from a recurrence of a Covid-19 pandemic of this magnitude. However, Covid-19 will likely not go away when we do get a vaccine. First generation vaccines usually are not able to stop a new virus in its tracks. It may not prevent you from getting infected but may help keep you out of the hospital or from getting a severe form of the infection. It may be future generations of the vaccines that will target more of the virus and, hopefully, generate longer lasting immunity than the first vaccines will offer. Even with some companies already producing vaccine, there won't be enough supply to manage a global pandemic. We will need to distribute the vaccine globally and prioritize who in the U.S. gets the initial doses. If we are not able to provide millions of doses of vaccine then we will not be able to reach the herd immunity that will be necessary to prevent widespread outbreaks. Two of the leading manufactured vaccines (Oxford University and the U.S. biotech firm Moderna) will likely require two doses *(App 13-15 Ref.)*. This doubles the number of doses to treat a large population of 328 million in the U.S. Even once the vaccines are available, the SARS-CoV-2 virus may still be infecting us, although the numbers of infections and deaths will likely be lower.

You should prepare as best you can in case the vaccines are not the end of SARS-CoV-2 virus. Take a serious look at implementing the anti-inflammatory diet and incorporating exercise into your lifestyle. No matter what happens, you will be healthier and likely live longer.

14 CLINICAL EXPERIENCE WITH THE ANTI-INFLAMMATORY DIET

As I mentioned at the outset, I am a facial plastic and reconstructive surgeon who performs primarily aesthetic and functional rhinoplasty. I was initially trained as an otolaryngologist (ENT) and went on to study facial plastic and reconstructive surgery. You may ask, why am I interested in the anti-inflammatory diet, comorbidities and the Covid-19 pandemic? First of all, I am a physician first and foremost. I spend a lot of time talking to patients about their nasal, facial and total body problems. I explain how the anti-inflammatory diet can speed along their postoperative recovery and also help them manage their nasal allergies. Many times I am counseling them on their other ailments such as back pain, joint pain, arthritis, rosacea, acne and even asthma and other comorbidities, and I will give them guidance on how the diet can help their symptoms. In a way, I have become more of a holistic doctor as well as a facial plastic surgeon.

Skin cancers

I treat a lot of patients with skin cancers, doing the reconstructions after the skin cancers are removed. Many of my patients have had multiple skin cancers, with new ones popping up every couple of years. This is due to chronic sun exposure and sunburns back when they were younger. It is very discouraging for patients when they keep developing these recurrent skin cancers. I explain to them that their diet is important in the development of their skin cancers. I explain that they have damaged skin cells and that free radicals in their body attack their skin cells and ultimately trigger skin cancers (Figure 22). I discuss how decreasing their body's free radicals can help to decrease further skin cancer formation. This can be achieved by implementing an anti-inflammatory diet and taking supplements such as green tea and curcumin with bioperine, which can inhibit squamous cell skin cancer[181] as well as other skin cancers.[182] I also discuss types of sunscreens to use and how to employ skin cancer prevention measures such as the anti-inflammatory diet and green tea.

Nasal and sinus allergies

The inflammation of the nasal and sinus mucosa that makes your nose stuffy or blocks your sinus opening is triggered by your immune system's response to allergens or other environmental factors. This inflammatory response is accentuated even further with the intake of inflammatory foods such as sugars and simple carbohydrates. I believe the most effective way to solve your problems with nasal and sinus disease is to decrease the inflammation in your nasal and sinus mucosa through the anti-inflammatory diet, proper supplements and exercise. This is the "cure your nose and sinuses program," which is a wellness-based lifestyle. As my patients experienced, you can dramatically improve your nasal and sinus symptoms by keeping track of everything that you eat and drink. Follow the program as we have described and monitor your progress.

I wanted to show how the anti-inflammatory diet can help to blunt a patient's response to allergens. In a clinical study we enrolled patients with moderate to severe nasal allergies to a four-month protocol. Patients initially had blood work drawn, had their BMI measured and underwent a thorough intranasal examination looking at the appearance of the nasal mucosa. Preoperative baseline symptoms and extent of compromise were recorded during the history and documented in extensive pre-study questionnaires.

During the first month of the study patients were asked to eat their normal diet, recording everything they ate or drank. Additionally, they recorded their nasal symptoms and rated them on a nasal symptom scale that could be quantified.[183] All of this information was recorded in a diary that they kept. At the beginning of the second month of the study the patients were asked to go on the anti-inflammatory diet. Clear instructions were given on what they should eat and what they should avoid. Reference materials were provided as well as green tea, fish oil and high-quality extra virgin olive oil. Patients were asked to drink a minimum of two glasses of green tea a day and use the olive oil in cooking and in their foods. They took the fish oil capsules as directed as well.

The study showed that during the second through the fourth months the patients found a significant improvement in their nasal symptoms when they were compliant with the diet. They also noted that when they ate inflammatory foods their symptoms worsened. Most of the patients noted that their noses became stuffy with increased drainage soon after eating inflammatory foods. Additionally, the following morning they would wake up with increased nasal drainage and stuffiness. One of the most beneficial aspects of the study was that the patients became educated on the anti-inflammatory diet and they came to know what foods made their symptoms worse. This knowledge is very important because it gives patients the power to make their dietary choices based on how their own body will react to allergens. Many of the patients continue the diet to this day.

Interestingly, many of the patients lost weight during the study and also felt much better overall. Those who had arthritis, rosacea, generalized back pain and other inflammatory disorders felt improvement in their symptoms. Many patients slept better and had more energy. Most of the patients also noted a dramatic improvement in the appearance of their skin. Their skin was clearer, with fewer blemishes and with better tone and coloration. Blood work showed a trend toward improvement in high-density lipoproteins (HDL) and lowering of low-density lipoproteins (LDL) and triglycerides. Total cholesterol was decreased as well. C-reactive protein, which measures total body inflammation, was reduced in most patients. The patients who were the most compliant had the most consistent improvement in their symptoms.

The indications for sinus surgery require a diagnosis of chronic rhinosinusitis (CRS). Chronic rhinosinusitis is the underlying disorder that is linked to the allergies and inflammation. A task force convened by the American Academy of Otolaryngology-Head & Neck Surgery in 1997 would define CRS based on six major and seven minor symptoms, including facial pressure/pain, nasal obstruction, and nasal discharge as major symptoms and cough, headache, fatigue, dental pain, and ear pain/pressure/fullness as minor symptoms.[184] A patient needed two or three of these symptoms for at least three months to have a "strong clinical history" for CRS and one or two for a "possible diagnosis." It has been calculated that 12.5% of Americans have CRS[185] and 10.9% of Europeans.[186] Based on these numbers, a very large percentage of patients with allergic rhinitis would have chronic rhinosinusitis and could be candidates for sinus surgery. Most patients with allergies and chronic rhinosinusitis can usually be treated effectively with antibiotics and a short course of steroids. The steroids would decrease the inflammation in the sinuses and allow the openings to the sinuses to open up to allow drainage and resolution of the infection.

The inflammation of the nasal and sinus mucosa that makes your nose stuffy or blocks your sinus opening is triggered by your immune system's response to allergens or other environmental factors. This inflammatory response is accentuated even further with the intake of inflammatory foods such as sugars, simple carbohydrates, etc. Chronic rhinosinusitis is the underlying disorder that is linked to the allergies and inflammation. I believe the most effective way to solve your problems with nasal and sinus disease is to decrease the inflammation in your nasal and sinus mucosa through the anti-inflammatory diet, proper supplements and exercise.

Anti-inflammatory diet and rhinoplasty

My clinical practice is primarily aesthetic and functional rhinoplasty. After rhinoplasty, patients will tend to have significant swelling and some bruising. Additionally, their nasal breathing may be blocked due to swelling on the inside of their nose. I have found it to be very helpful for patients if they adhere to a low-salt, anti-inflammatory diet after surgery. The low salt intake of less than 1000 milligrams per day helps to keep the swelling down. I have also noted that when patients eat inflammatory foods their nose will tend to be more inflamed and swollen. They may have increased redness of the skin of their nose and increased stuffiness. I frequently tell patients to adhere to an anti-inflammatory diet to decrease their nasal inflammation, decrease swelling and improve their nasal breathing. Patients who tend to have seasonal allergies or rosacea are most prone to experiencing increased swelling after eating inflammatory foods. Specific foods that should be avoided include dairy products, sugars, simple carbohydrates (pasta, rice and breads) and corn products. Foods that are high in saturated fats also tend to make the nose swell up. I will also have patients drink two cups of green tea per day. Having a cup of matcha green tea is even better for decreasing inflammation.

When I see patients in the office whose noses are swollen, I frequently ask them what they ate for dinner the night before. Typically, they had an inflammatory food item or a salty meal. In some cases, I will ask them to keep a diary of their food intake and also rate their nose swelling and nasal stuffiness. This exercise will allow them to identify particularly problematic foods.

Alcohol will also tend to increase inflammation and nasal swelling externally and internally. Patients will frequently experience nasal stuffiness soon after having an alcoholic beverage. I tell patients to limit their alcohol intake to one drink and to avoid sugary drinks and red or white wines.

I have found it beneficial to put patients on an anti-inflammatory diet for most facial surgeries, including eyelid surgery, facelift surgery and facial fat grafting. Healing after any type of skin resurfacing (laser or chemical peel) will also be improved on the anti-inflammatory diet.

The anti-inflammatory diet and some anti-inflammatory supplements can help patients recovering from surgery *(App 14-1 Ref.)*.[187] Decreasing the inflammation in the body may also help to control pain postoperatively *(App 14-2 Ref.)*. Patients can also take some supplements such as curcumin and vitamin C. Curcumin has been shown to help attenuate postoperative pain after surgery.[188]

Eating well after surgery and staying well hydrated are critical to maximizing healing. This is particularly important after nasal and facial surgery. Decreasing inflammation and bolstering the immune system are very important to build your defenses after nasal surgery to prevent infection from SARS-CoV-2. This is particularly important during these times when this novel coronavirus is a potential threat.

Monitoring your progress

It is important to monitor your progress on the anti-inflammatory diet. This can be accomplished by recording your symptoms on a daily basis. You will need to record everything that you eat and drink and also record your nasal symptoms as well as other general body parameters such as allergy symptoms, back and joint pain, headache, stiffness, asthma symptoms, sleep patterns, alertness and general mood. You should also record the exercise that you are participating in and any supplements that you are taking and the quantities that you are using. These records will allow you to correlate how you feel in relation to your adherence to the anti-inflammatory diet. Try to accurately record your data for at least two months. This will give you adequate data to make some sound conclusions on where you stand with the program and how it has affected your quality of life. You should also monitor your blood pressure and body weight. A mechanism to record such data will be available in the near future via electronic app *(App 14-3 Ref. +)*.

The other major benefit of recording your data is that it will allow you to identify foods that are particularly deleterious to the state of your nose and sinuscs and general health. Typically, patients will complain of nasal stuffiness, nasal drainage and obstructed nasal breathing when they wake up in the morning. If patients track back to the day before, they likely ate some inflammatory foods or drank some inflammatory fluids. Unfortunately, many people are married to their inflammatory "feel good" foods. What we will typically do is eat inflammatory foods and then treat the subsequent symptoms with medications. By doing this we are just managing the symptoms and not correcting the underlying problem. The underlying problem is the foods we eat and drink.

In order to implement this diet you will likely need to make some lifestyle changes. This will involve changing your approach to food and food choices. If you think of your food and drink as the direct link to your overall health, you can rationalize the importance of making some changes. If you additionally link the inflammatory foods to not feeling well, this can be the biggest impetus to making the changes. Another important factor is the long-term effects of inflammation on your body. Years of inflammation will result in developing many chronic diseases such as heart disease, diabetes, arthritis, cancer, and autoimmune disorders such as lupus. If you are constantly getting skin cancers, it may be time to do something about it.

When you start on the anti-inflammatory diet, you should measure your waistline at the outset, as explained in Chapter 7. An excellent method to measure your waist is to take the measurement at the intersection of the top of the ilium (hip bone) and a vertical line from the center of the armpit.(Figure 23) The primary reason is to monitor your progress and see if your visceral fat is decreasing on the diet. You should do the measurement once every two weeks to monitor changes in the girth of your midsection. If you are strict on the anti-inflammatory diet, you will likely see a decrease in the circumference of your stomach area. This would also likely indicate that you are losing some visceral fat. This is a good indication that you are doing the right things with your diet. Another good indicator is some weight loss associated with the diet. Most people who go on the diet could lose a significant amount of weight, mostly in the midsection of their body. This is by far the most important area to lose fat. This is a good consequence of the diet and can continue while you stick to it. Changes on the AI-keto diet will be even more dramatic with greater weight loss and a greater reduction in your waistline measurement. (Figure 24)

I have many patients who went on the anti-inflammatory diet. Many have noted the improvement in their nasal and sinus symptoms and their general health. Some of their experiences are noted in the next chapter.

15
PATIENT EXPERIENCES WITH THE ANTI-INFLAMMATORY DIET

Patient testimonials

Patient A

After struggling with nose pain inexplicably at different times several months after my surgery I had an "aha!" moment with Dr. Toriumi when he connected the dots between sugar and simple carbs and my nose pain. After Dr Toriumi explained to me how the carbs caused inflammation in my nose, I began keeping track and clearly saw the direct result of managing my sugar and carb intake and any nose/sinus issues. I am so grateful to Dr Toriumi!

Patient B

I have had allergy and sinus problems my entire life. I usually have to take at least two medications to treat my allergies and even with these medications I still am miserable at times. Dr. Toriumi has been my doctor for years and he has worked with me to help me with my problems. He told me about the anti-inflammatory diet years ago. I was very interested and read a lot on the subject. I read some of the references that he gave me and found them very informative. The basic program was to stop eating the simple carbohydrates and sweets. In the past, I would have a lot of carbohydrates such as bagels, potatoes, pasta and rice. I also ate a lot of chips and bread. I had a very strong liking for carbs. With the reading and after listening to Dr. Toriumi, I started to avoid the simple carbohydrates and found that I felt better and my nasal symptoms decreased. I found that if I ate a simple carbohydrate, my nose would stuff up and I would start to clear my throat. It was an amazing association that was very clear. If I avoided the simple carbohydrates I had minimal if any nasal symptoms and I generally felt better. I also exercise several times a week. If I worked out and had carbs the same day I would be more sore the next day. I also started drinking green tea and found that to be very helpful. In fact, I now drink at least two cups of green tea a day. Now that I am on this diet I know what to do if I need to feel good. I do cheat occasionally, and I can tell the difference. So I choose when I would like to cheat. With the Covid-19 pandemic and lockdown, I have been cheating a bit more but still know when I need to avoid the bad stuff. Thank you Dr. Toriumi for clueing me in on the anti-inflammatory diet.

Patient C

I have been a patient of Dr. Toriumi for many years. He has treated me for my skin cancers for years. I had a lot of sun exposure over the years and suffered many sunburns as a child. Unfortunately, this has resulted in recurring skin cancers. I get them taken off too frequently. Dr. Toriumi has repaired many of them. He told me to go onto the anti-inflammatory diet to help slow the growth of these cancers. He also told me to start some curcumin and green tea. Since making these changes my skin cancers are coming less often. Another big benefit has been the improvement in my general health. I can tell when I have eaten something inflammatory as I have worsening of my body pains and my rosacea gets worse. My skin looks terrible if I eat bad foods. I still like carbs and sweet things and those are the ones that make everything worse. It is very difficult to be good all the time and when I cheat on the diet I pay the consequences. I thank Dr. Toriumi for giving me the information about the diet. It has helped me tremendously.

Patient D

I never had an issue with my weight or my appearance. I was an active 40 year old who maintained a good weight. Then I was diagnosed with an autoimmune disease that required use of high dose steroids. After my diagnosis, I gained weight, and due to the steroids, my face had the appearance of a "moon face." Additionally, I had corrective surgery that left me with postoperative swelling. These issues persisted even after ceasing the use of oral steroids and exercising. I still had approximately 15 pounds that, even with exercise, I was unable to lose and I had joint discomfort.

I strictly followed Dr. Toriumi's advice and diet for four weeks. I ate lean meats (chicken, pork and salmon) with vegetables. No sugar, red meat, carbohydrates, salt or dairy. Additionally, I drank copious amounts of water and green tea. I drank daily at least four cups of green tea, with two tea bags in each cup.

Due to strict adherence to his advice and dietary suggestions; at the end of the four weeks I had lost 14 pounds and believe the diet reduced the appearance of the "moon face" and reduced swelling. I had less joint discomfort and my skin looked healthier.

After the initial four weeks I began to moderately indulge in different foods. I continue to follow his advice and drink green tea every day, which has helped me to maintain my weight.

Patient E

My name is Lakeshia.L. I would like to talk about my inflamed diet. Dr. Toriumi has been talking to me for years about changing my diet! And I'm hoping that after reading his book it will give me the motivation I need to get in gear! I'm a lover of Gino's East pizza, Mexican food and just about anything that's fried. I love very sweet sparkling wine and beer. On any given day, I'll drink a bottle of wine topped off by a 16-ounce can of light beer. I will add ketchup to just about anything I eat. My grandmother passed away at the age of 62 of a heart attack, and her diet certainly played a very big role in that. With my unhealthy eating, I've developed high blood pressure and various other health issues. I'm excited to read Dr. Toriumi's new *book on the anti- inflammatory diet, including the recipes and any other advice for a healthier lifestyle.*

Patient F

I cannot say enough about Dr. Dean Toriumi! After my rhinoplasty surgery with him last month, he suggested an anti-inflammatory and low sodium food diet. It only took about a week for cravings to go away and I have truly felt a significant difference in my energy levels and mood. I was surprised to find out that it wasn't hard to eat more strictly. With his guidance and knowledge about certain foods, I can maintain a healthy and balanced diet by eating more fresh fruits, vegetables, and other foods that have healthy fats.

Patient G

About six months ago I met with Dr. Dean Toriumi to try and fix my nose, which has bothered me my whole life after multiple nose injuries. I have had surgeries to correct the problem, but they just ended up making things worse. I looked horrible, I could not breath, and I had pretty much given up hope and accepted that I'd just live the rest of my life like this rather than trying to have another surgery and possibly make it even worse (which every doctor told me would probably happen) No doctor would take my case. So after lots of research and hearing all the hype about Dr. Toriumi, I said all right, one last try. What do I have to lose at this point?

Meeting with him was a completely different experience. He looked at me, addressed the issues and told me no problem, we'll fix it. He was extremely confident that he could take care of this complex case (that no the doctor would touch) with no problem...

I'm writing this now six months post-surgery, and he did exactly as he said he would. He repaired my breathing, my aesthetic and my self-esteem. He has exceeded my expectations more than I ever could have imagined. I was looking for improvement, but he gave me perfection.

As far as the healing process, he suggested a low-sodium, anti-inflammatory diet, which I thought was interesting at first. This will help my nose? Huh? But I wanted to do everything I could to get the best outcome, so I followed his suggestions and switched to a diet consisting of lots of green tea; good fruits like berries and apples; vegetables; egg whites; chicken breast; lean ground turkey; beans; a daily spinach salad with olive oil, avocado and nuts; and foods high in omega-3s.

This diet worked so amazingly for me that I still stick to it (and enjoy it!). Not only do I feel it significantly helped the healing process, but it has made me feel amazing physically and mentally. I love it.

I feel great, I look great, and thanks to Dr. T I'm now more excited and motivated about life.

Thank you, thank you, thank you, Dr. Toriumi!

Patient H

Although I had always considered myself to be a "healthy eater" and have taken good care of myself, I had continuous sinus issues that I could not seem to get a handle on – stuffiness, difficulty breathing during exercise, poor sleep, and seasonal allergies. When Dr. Toriumi enrolled me in his anti-inflammatory study, I wasn't certain that it was going to make that much difference beyond that of my normal diet, given that I was otherwise healthy, active and believed to be eating in that manner already. However, through tracking my intake and religiously adding the anti-inflammatory foods, it quickly become clear that my current diet included more inflammatory items than I previously realized, and they were indeed contributing to many of my issues. I participated in the study primarily over the summer months, and quite naturally, some days my adherence was better than others, particularly on weekends. It quickly became clear that the correlation between diligently eliminating inflammatory foods and how I felt day to day were intricately linked as I saw my respiratory ailments diminish when I was most diligent. To this day I continue to follow the diet, although I have since added matcha tea in addition to traditional green tea, and even carry packets with me to drink in place of coffee. The other pleasant 'side effect' of this diet was that I naturally lost weight and gained more energy in the process. Having eaten this way for a few years now, I have been able to eliminate my nasal spray and feel better than ever. I am very grateful to Dr. Toriumi for including me in the study and teaching me how to take control of my health and wellness.

Additional testimonials can be found on the website toriumidiet.com.

16
FINAL THOUGHTS: LEARNING TO LIVE WITH COVID-19

In the era of Covid-19 we will need to live differently and make changes in how we move forward. It is likely that hand-shaking and hugging will be practiced less. Social distancing will likely become the norm. We will see people wearing masks and gloves. Our hands will be constantly dry from frequent hand washing. Airplanes will have more empty seats. Stadiums will have fewer spectators. Massive gatherings such as outdoor concerts will likely be discouraged or at least regulated. Many more people will work from home and more children will be homeschooled. Even if most of these changes are just temporary, if a new pandemic comes, these restrictions will likely be reestablished.

However, there are some positives. Families have come closer together. Parents have spent more time with their children. Many people have become more dependent on their faith. You can look at this as an opportunity to improve your diet and curb or eliminate some of your comorbidities and better prepare yourself for the next potential pandemic. Even if it never comes, you will be less inflamed, you will feel better and look better, and you will be a healthier person better equipped to fight any virus. No matter what the future brings, our health will likely become more important to withstanding the infectious threats to our lives.

Eat anti-inflammatory to live less inflamed.
Dean M. Toriumi, MD.

Index

A

Acetone breath 91
Acne xix, 79, 102, 103, 104, 174
Acute respiratory distress syndrome (ARDS) xix, 69
Adult onset diabetes xvi
AI-keto diet xii, xiii, 162, 181, 207
Allergies v, 4, 5, 7, 8, 174, 175, 176, 177, 178, 183, 187
Almond butter 24, 27, 111, 129, 130, 132, 133, 137, 138, 152, 156
Almond butter ball 156
Almond milk 20, 131, 137, 139, 140, 150, 159
Almonds 22, 26, 87, 129, 132, 140, 145, 152, 155
Alzheimer's disease 47, 62, 75, 215
Antibodies 5, 7, 9, 202
Antibody 7
Anti-inflammatory diet v, vi, vii, viii, x, xi, xii, xiii, xvi, xvii, 7, 8, 14, 15, 22, 24, 28, 35, 41, 43, 45, 50, 52, 60, 70, 78, 81, 83, 84, 87, 88, 90, 92, 93, 94, 95, 97, 102, 103, 106, 108, 109, 111, 112, 113, 114, 116, 117, 119, 128, 136, 144, 152, 153, 162, 166, 167, 168, 171, 172, 174, 175, 176, 177, 178, 179, 180, 181, 183, 184, 187, 207
Anti-inflammatory diet with keto-push 97
Anti-inflammatory foods vi, xii, xvi, xix, 29, 36, 89, 108, 113, 162, 187
Antioxidants 21, 30, 33, 36, 48, 56, 60, 66, 125, 205, 214
Apple cider vinegar 16, 26, 92, 93, 94, 155, 160
Apples 14, 144
Arthritis xix, 24, 38, 46, 54, 60, 63, 65, 66, 103, 106, 107, 108, 165, 174, 176, 180, 216
Artichoke 27, 30, 31, 32, 144, 147, 154, 160, 203
Asparagus 27, 28, 39, 81, 87, 89, 112, 115, 129, 138, 144, 149, 154, 159
Asthma v, xi, xv, xvi, 164, 168, 174, 179
Atherosclerosis 15, 51, 214
Avocados 50, 94, 95

B

Back pain v, vii, 16, 54, 106, 108, 109, 174, 176
Bacon xi, 33, 87, 93, 114, 115
Bagels 15, 183
Balsamic vinegar 16, 23, 27, 42, 47, 48, 49, 89, 93, 111, 129, 130, 135, 137, 139, 140, 145, 146, 147, 149, 153, 155, 157, 161, 214
Bananas 19, 21
Barbecue 29, 35
Beef 33, 40, 81, 112, 121, 132, 133, 212
Black rice 122, 123, 136, 150
Blueberries 19, 33, 41, 50, 65, 88, 94, 125, 129, 136, 137, 139, 140, 144, 145, 146, 147, 149, 150, 151, 154, 157, 159
Blue zones 82, 219, 222

Body mass index 12
Brain 12, 42, 57, 62, 68, 70, 72, 75, 85, 91, 92, 93, 96, 97, 212, 221
Brain derived neurotrophic factor (BDNF) 72
Brain fog 91
Bread 14, 16, 23, 24, 42, 50, 85, 87, 94, 103, 111, 112, 120, 133, 134, 135, 136, 138, 139, 140, 141, 144, 148, 149, 150, 151, 152, 154, 155, 157, 160, 183, 211
Breakfast vi, 15, 24, 66, 120, 152, 153
Broccoli vi, 14, 25, 26, 28, 29, 30, 33, 39, 40, 50, 81, 87, 88, 112, 113, 115, 121, 132, 135, 144, 145, 154, 155, 157, 169
Brown rice 136, 142
Butter 24, 27, 51, 52, 87, 111, 114, 120, 129, 130, 132, 133, 135, 137, 138, 149, 150, 152, 156, 160

C

Caffeine 21, 55, 56, 57, 58, 59, 204
Caffeine effect 21, 56, 57, 204
Cancer 19, 20, 24, 32, 33, 41, 46, 48, 54, 56, 58, 60, 61, 66, 77, 79, 115, 116, 123, 165, 169, 174, 180, 211, 213, 216, 221
Capsaicin 38, 212
Carbohydrates 13, 14, 16, 25, 26, 27, 28, 33, 42, 48, 81, 85, 86, 87, 88, 89, 92, 102, 103, 112, 120, 121, 124, 128, 144, 152, 153, 154, 170, 175, 177, 178, 183, 185, 207, 211
Cardiovascular disease xv, 12, 65, 77, 93, 211, 216, 217, 219, 220
Carrots 26, 27, 28, 39, 40, 50, 111, 124, 137, 149
Cauliflower 28, 29, 30, 33, 37, 81, 87, 88, 112, 113, 115, 129, 130, 136, 142, 144, 146, 154, 156, 159, 160, 169
Celery 26, 27, 39, 156
Chamomile tea 137, 141, 145, 151, 156
Chamomile teas 58
Cheese xi, 20, 22, 23, 33, 37, 112, 115, 120, 122, 129, 130, 131, 132, 133, 135, 137, 138, 140, 148, 150, 151, 158
Cherries 33, 41
Chia seeds 19, 20, 81, 89, 139, 145, 146, 150, 154, 157, 161
Chicken 22, 34, 35, 81, 120, 121, 131, 137, 148, 155
Chicken breast 24, 35, 94, 114, 120, 130, 145, 146, 155, 187
Chicken soup 159
Chicken tacos 131
Chili 23, 25, 26, 50, 51, 121, 123, 150, 156
Cholesterol 18, 19, 20, 31, 48, 50, 51, 93, 123, 176
Cigarettes 16
Coconut milk 113
Coffee 18, 21, 55, 57, 59, 101, 102, 139, 142, 143, 145, 146, 147, 148, 188, 204
Colitis 65
Colon cancer 19, 20, 115
Comorbidities xv, xvi, xx, 10, 12, 13, 16, 54, 59, 62, 75, 77, 78, 86, 95, 104, 119, 144, 162, 164, 165, 166, 167, 168, 174, 188, 210, 222
Cooking 8, 35, 40, 45, 47, 49, 50, 111, 113, 121, 125, 171, 176
Core exercises 73, 95, 109, 154
Corn 14, 18, 23, 27, 33, 34, 35, 50, 112, 120, 136, 144, 154, 178
Corn syrup 14, 23, 27, 35

Corticosteroids x
Cortisol 43, 70, 75, 79, 80, 83, 170, 171, 218
Couscous 14, 32, 115, 136
Covid-19 i, iii, iv, v, vi, vii, viii, ix, x, xi, xiii, xv, xvi, xvii, xix, xx, 1, 2, 4, 9, 10, 12, 13, 16, 43, 59, 67, 69, 70, 71, 72, 75, 77, 78, 83, 118, 119, 144, 162, 163, 164, 165, 166, 168, 169, 170, 171, 172, 174, 184, 188, 210, 211, 216, 217, 222
C-reactive protein 68, 116, 176, 216
Cream cheese 122, 150
Curcumin vi, 58, 60, 61, 62, 66, 108, 109, 174, 179, 184, 215, 223

D

Dairy 20, 22, 23, 24, 25, 26, 27, 32, 40, 87, 115, 122, 124, 128, 158, 178, 185
Death rates xv
Decaffeinated green tea 19, 21, 55, 140, 145, 146
Dehydration 81, 101, 117
Dementia 79, 96, 165
Depression xvii, 70, 72, 79, 96, 97, 118, 170, 220
Diabetes v, vii, ix, xi, xv, xvi, 12, 13, 14, 15, 16, 48, 49, 54, 56, 60, 65, 77, 82, 86, 95, 103, 119, 164, 165, 167, 168, 180, 217, 219
Diet iv, v, vi, vii, viii, x, xi, xii, xiii, xvi, xvii, xix, 7, 8, 12, 14, 15, 16, 19, 20, 21, 22, 23, 24, 26, 28, 29, 30, 32, 33, 35, 39, 41, 42, 43, 45, 46, 47, 48, 49, 50, 51, 52, 54, 59, 60, 61, 62, 66, 69, 70, 78, 80, 81, 82, 83, 84, 85, 86, 87, 88, 89, 90, 91, 92, 93, 94, 95, 96, 97, 99, 100, 102, 103, 106, 107, 108, 109, 111, 112, 113, 114, 116, 117, 119, 124, 125, 128, 136, 144, 145, 152, 153, 162, 165, 166, 167, 168, 171, 172, 174, 175, 176, 177, 178, 179, 180, 181, 183, 184, 185, 186, 187, 188, 207, 214, 216, 220
Dinner vi, 26, 27, 28, 33, 40, 42, 81, 88, 94, 111, 129, 131, 133, 134, 137, 138, 140, 150, 152, 153, 178

E

Edamame 26, 39, 51, 80, 112, 115, 123, 138
Egg bites 134
Eggs 13, 18, 22, 39, 51, 111, 120, 122, 132, 140, 141, 143, 147, 149, 152, 157, 160
Egg white protein 19, 20, 81, 145, 146, 150, 157
Egg whites 94, 161, 187
Elderly 165, 166, 219
Electrolytes 91, 101, 102, 135, 137, 138, 143, 148, 149, 150, 158, 161
Endorphins 70, 72
Energy bars 27
Epigenetics 167, 222
Epinephrine 68
Estrogen 79
Exercise v, vi, 12, 16, 24, 43, 68, 69, 70, 71, 72, 74, 75, 77, 80, 83, 106, 165, 166, 167, 168, 170, 172, 175, 177, 178, 179, 183, 185, 187, 212, 217
Extra-virgin olive oil 23, 45, 46, 47, 48, 49, 50, 51, 89, 94, 138, 153, 213
Ezekiel bread 24, 50, 111, 120, 138, 139, 140, 141, 148, 149, 151, 152

F

Fajitas 137

Family 13, 43, 57, 82, 124
Farm raised 36
Fast food 119, 120, 121
Fasting xvi, 12, 86, 153, 155, 156, 159, 161, 165
Fatigue 5, 79, 95, 107, 118, 177, 223
Fat loss 83, 86, 91, 99
Fiber 19, 20, 22, 30, 41, 66, 86, 88, 94, 112, 115, 116, 123, 125, 169
Fish 13, 22, 24, 29, 36, 37, 38, 39, 42, 62, 63, 64, 65, 66, 81, 89, 94, 114, 122, 123, 124, 144, 150, 175, 176, 212, 215
Flaxseed 157, 211
Folate 31, 66, 123
Free radicals 32, 60, 61, 66, 69, 174, 205
Friends 43, 82
Fructose 13, 14, 23, 27, 35
Fruit 13, 14, 19, 21, 41, 50, 66, 88, 115, 116, 139, 140, 154
Fuji apples 41

G

Gamma aminobutyric acid (GABA) 96
Garbanzo beans 22, 26, 29, 33, 125
Garlic 23, 24, 26, 28, 30, 31, 32, 35, 38, 40, 48, 50, 112, 113, 114, 125, 129, 138, 139, 140, 141, 146, 147, 148, 151, 160, 211
Ghee 51, 52
Ginger 21, 26, 40, 57, 80, 93, 113, 135, 139, 142, 143, 146, 147, 148, 149, 157, 215
Ginger tea 139, 142, 146, 147, 149, 157
Glucose 12, 13, 14, 15, 49, 71, 85, 90, 96, 103, 153, 202
Glycemic index (GI) 13
Grains 41, 124
Grass-fed 33, 34, 81, 112, 131
Greek chicken 158
Green beans 28, 30, 40, 81, 87, 88, 89, 112, 115, 120, 140, 144, 151, 154, 161
Green tea vi, 19, 21, 50, 54, 55, 56, 57, 58, 59, 66, 81, 88, 94, 103, 108, 123, 124, 128, 129, 130, 131, 132, 133, 134, 135, 136, 137, 138, 139, 140, 141, 142, 143, 144, 145, 146, 147, 148, 149, 150, 151, 154, 155, 156, 157, 158, 159, 160, 161, 174, 175, 176, 178, 184, 185, 187, 188, 214, 215, 219
Grilled broccoli 135, 145, 155
Grilled chicken 114, 120, 125, 137, 155
Grilled fish 114
Grilled salmon 139, 143, 147
Grilled salmon 129
Guacamole 94, 155, 156, 157, 159, 161

H

Hard-boiled eggs 22, 143, 149, 152, 157
Heavy metals 22
Hemoglobin A1c 12, 49
Hemp protein 143
High-density lipoprotein 83

High-density lipoproteins 63, 176
High fructose corn syrup 14, 23, 27, 35
High-glycemic 13, 14, 15, 16, 23, 103
Honey 13, 25, 40
Honeydew 159
Hot dogs 33
Hummus 25, 26, 27, 111, 120, 129, 137, 141, 143, 149
Hydration 99, 220
Hydration 101
Hypertension v, xv, 66, 95, 108, 119, 164, 167, 221

I

Ice cream 36, 41, 109, 124, 129, 132
Immune response xix, 6, 9, 165
Immune senescence 166
Immune system v, vi, x, xi, xiii, xviii, xx, 5, 6, 7, 8, 9, 10, 58, 68, 71, 82, 103, 106, 118, 119, 166, 175, 177, 179, 201, 214, 221
Immunity xvi, 24, 123, 172, 221
Inflammaging 165, 208
Inflammation iv, v, x, xi, xvii, xviii, xix, xx, 5, 7, 8, 18, 20, 22, 24, 25, 36, 39, 45, 46, 51, 56, 58, 59, 62, 63, 66, 68, 69, 70, 71, 72, 75, 80, 83, 91, 96, 97, 102, 103, 106, 107, 108, 109, 116, 125, 129, 144, 151, 165, 166, 167, 169, 170, 175, 176, 177, 178, 179, 180, 183, 208, 210, 211, 212, 214, 215, 217, 220
Inflammatory foods vi, xi, xii, xvi, xix, 8, 10, 29, 36, 60, 82, 89, 97, 107, 108, 109, 113, 162, 165, 175, 176, 177, 178, 180, 187, 188
Interleukins 97

J

Jalapeño pepper 38
Japanese food 122, 123
Joints v, xviii, 46, 103, 106, 107, 109, 143
Juice 16, 21, 65, 66, 92, 142, 156, 216

K

Kale 21, 22, 27, 29, 30, 33, 80, 88, 89, 95, 131, 141, 144, 148, 151, 154, 155, 156, 158, 169
Kale chips 29, 131, 141, 148, 158
Ketchup 120, 185
Keto diet xi, xii, xiii, 52, 85, 86, 87, 88, 90, 91, 92, 93, 95, 153, 162, 181, 207
Ketones 85, 86, 89, 90, 91, 92, 93, 96
Keto push vi, vii, xii, xvii, 14, 15, 21, 22, 23, 24, 27, 28, 35, 81, 83, 84, 88, 89, 90, 91, 92, 93, 94, 95, 97, 100, 109, 111, 112, 113, 114, 116, 117, 120, 122, 128, 152, 153, 154, 162, 207
Ketosis 83, 85, 86, 87, 90, 93, 96, 153, 162, 219
Ketotic state 86, 88, 90, 91, 92, 93, 95, 153, 162
Kidney disease xi
Krill 36, 39, 65

L

Lethargy v, 7, 91
Leukocytes 71
Leukotrienes 97
Longevity 82
Low-density lipoproteins 176
Low glycemic 14, 211, 220
L-theanine 57
Lunch 22, 129, 130, 131, 132, 133, 134, 135, 137, 138, 139, 140, 141, 142, 143, 145, 146, 147, 148, 149, 150, 151, 155, 156, 157, 158, 159, 160, 161
Lungs ix, x, xix, 2, 9, 69, 71, 118
Lupus 54, 60, 103, 180, 220
Lymphocytes 6
Lymphoid organs 6

M

Mackerel 37, 64, 89, 94, 108, 122, 123, 150
Magnesium 22, 31, 95, 123, 125
Mahi mahi 37, 39
Maki 122
Maple syrup 14, 131
Masks 5, 170, 188
Mast cells 7, 202
Matcha 21, 55, 56, 57, 130, 133, 135, 136, 137, 138, 139, 140, 141, 143, 144, 145, 146, 147, 148, 149, 150, 154, 155, 156, 157, 158, 159, 160, 161, 178, 188, 205
Meal plans xii, 154, 162
Meditation 75, 218
Mediterranean diet xvi, 45, 46, 52, 89, 117
Melon 116
Memory 72, 116, 117
Memory loss 116
Mercury 22, 37, 38, 39, 63, 64, 65, 111, 122, 148, 150
Milk 20, 39, 51, 113, 131, 137, 139, 140, 150, 159
Miso 113, 123, 158, 221
Mitochondria 71, 165
Mood xi, xvii, 57, 70, 75, 96, 97, 118, 179, 186, 220
Mucosa 3, 4, 7, 175, 177
Muscle 20, 42, 58, 68, 70, 71, 73, 79, 86, 95, 218
Mustard 25, 129, 138, 141, 149

N

Nasal allergies 4, 7, 8, 174, 175
Nasal obstruction 2, 4, 7, 177
Nasal septum 2, 4
Nerves 5, 106
Nose v, vi, ix, xvii, xviii, xix, xx, 2, 3, 4, 5, 7, 10, 103, 143, 175, 177, 178, 180, 183, 186, 187, 200, 201

O

Oatmeal 14, 15, 19, 50, 55, 131, 135, 137, 145, 150, 159
Obesity v, ix, xi, xv, xvi, 12, 107, 164, 212, 217, 218
Okinawa diet xvi, 124, 125
Okinawan sweet potatoes 124, 125
Oleocanthal 45, 46, 47
Olive oil vi, 16, 23, 24, 26, 27, 28, 29, 30, 31, 32, 33, 34, 35, 38, 39, 40, 42, 45, 46, 47, 48, 49, 50, 51, 52, 88, 89, 94, 111, 112, 113, 114, 115, 120, 125, 129, 130, 131, 133, 135, 137, 138, 139, 140, 141, 143, 145, 146, 147, 148, 149, 150, 151, 153, 154, 155, 157, 158, 160, 161, 176, 187, 213, 214
Olives 25, 47, 120, 129, 140, 160
Omega-3 fatty acids 18, 19, 22, 34, 36, 37, 39, 42, 62, 63, 64, 65, 89, 94, 95, 108, 123, 153
Omega-6 fatty acids 18, 20, 34, 36, 62, 63, 114
Omelet 130, 151, 158
Organic 16, 19, 33, 34, 37, 41, 81, 94, 112, 131, 133, 136, 137, 142, 144, 151, 154, 160
Osteoarthritis 46, 54
Ostia 2, 7

P

Pain v, vii, xvii, 3, 7, 16, 24, 38, 43, 51, 54, 58, 66, 75, 106, 107, 108, 109, 174, 176, 177, 179, 183, 221, 223
Parmesan cheese 130
Pasta 15, 16, 19, 23, 42, 85, 103, 113, 115, 129, 136, 141, 144, 154, 178, 183
Peach 135, 143, 148
Peanuts 26, 65, 87
Pepper 23, 26, 30, 35, 38, 40, 48, 50, 51, 61, 62, 109, 112, 125, 145, 147, 148
Peppers 25, 30, 37, 38, 39, 112, 121, 130, 137, 148, 158
Pilates 75
Pistachios 22, 26, 134
Pizza 8, 37, 50, 109, 112, 130, 148, 185
Polyphenols 30, 41, 48, 54, 58, 65, 116, 123, 214, 215
Pomegranate 65, 66, 143
Pomegranate juice 65, 66
Pork 114, 115, 121, 123, 185
Postoperative pain 179
Potassium 28, 31, 37, 95, 125
Potato chips 26, 27, 129
Potatoes 14, 25, 26, 112, 115, 121, 124, 125, 135, 183
Prediabetic 12, 15, 16
Prostaglandins 63
Protein 2, 3, 18, 19, 20, 22, 24, 26, 27, 28, 29, 32, 33, 34, 35, 37, 39, 41, 42, 55, 66, 68, 81, 87, 88, 89, 100, 111, 112, 113, 115, 116, 123, 143, 145, 146, 150, 151, 152, 157, 176, 200, 207, 214, 217, 220
Protein bars 26
Protein shake 18, 19, 81, 111
Psoriasis 60, 102, 103, 106

Q

Quinoa 39, 112, 115, 140, 142

R

Red meat 33, 37, 87, 112, 114, 154, 185
Red pepper 26, 50, 51
Red snapper 38
Resveratrol 65, 216
Rhinitis 5, 177
Rhinoplasty v, vii, 174, 177, 186
Rhinosinusitis 176, 177, 210, 223
Rice 14, 16, 42, 85, 103, 112, 115, 121, 122, 123, 132, 134, 136, 142, 144, 145, 150, 151, 154, 158, 159, 160, 178, 183
Roast 31, 55, 135
Romaine lettuce 25, 158
Romaine lettuce 88
Rooibos tea 59
Rosacea xix, 102, 103, 174, 176, 178, 184, 220
Running 68, 70

S

Salad 16, 22, 23, 24, 27, 33, 37, 42, 45, 48, 81, 94, 111, 112, 115, 123, 129, 130, 134, 135, 137, 139, 140, 141, 142, 143, 145, 146, 147, 148, 149, 150, 151, 155, 156, 157, 158, 159, 160, 161, 187
Salad dressing 24, 45, 48, 160
Salmon 22, 35, 36, 37, 38, 50, 62, 64, 89, 94, 108, 112, 113, 115, 122, 123, 129, 138, 139, 143, 145, 147, 148, 150, 152, 156, 157, 158, 160, 185
Salt 23, 26, 28, 29, 30, 31, 32, 34, 35, 37, 38, 40, 48, 50, 94, 112, 123, 125, 131, 133, 135, 138, 139, 140, 142, 145, 146, 147, 148, 149, 150, 151, 155, 158, 160, 178, 185
Sardines 22, 64, 89, 108, 148
Sardines 37, 94
SARS-CoV-2 virus x, xv, xvi, xvii, 2, 3, 4, 5, 8, 9, 10, 71, 86, 118, 162, 164, 166, 167, 169, 172, 200
Sashimi 122, 150
Sausage 120, 130, 141, 147
Sausages 33, 93, 120
Seaweed 123, 150, 158
Seaweed salad 123, 150
Septoplasty 4
Sesame oil 40, 51, 138, 142, 214
Shake 18, 19, 20, 21, 29, 50, 55, 66, 81, 88, 94, 111, 145, 146, 150, 151, 157
Sinuses xvii, xix, xx, 2, 3, 4, 7, 175, 177, 180, 200
Skin v, xvii, xix, 32, 34, 35, 38, 41, 43, 58, 66, 81, 99, 100, 101, 102, 103, 104, 106, 114, 117, 121, 125, 144, 151, 154, 174, 176, 178, 180, 184, 185, 207, 208, 220, 222
Skin cancer 58, 174
Skin cancers 32, 100, 174, 180, 184

Sleep xi, 58, 70, 79, 80, 81, 82, 92, 99, 117, 118, 119, 165, 179, 187, 221
Smell 2, 4, 5, 9
Smoking 16, 99
Snacks 26, 50, 66, 136, 155
Snacks 26
Sodium 28, 95, 101, 115, 116, 186, 187
Soup 25, 26, 40, 42, 43, 51, 113, 115, 121, 123, 125, 131, 132, 135, 138, 150, 158, 159
Soy 20, 37, 39, 40, 51, 80, 112, 124, 148, 159, 211
Soybeans 39, 115, 123
Soybeans 39
Soy milk 39, 159
Soy protein 20
Spatchcock chicken 34
Spinach vi, 21, 22, 27, 28, 30, 33, 56, 88, 112, 113, 133, 138, 139, 141, 144, 151, 154, 187
Steel cut oatmeal 14, 131, 135, 137, 150
Steroids 8, 177, 184, 185
Stew 40, 133, 159
Strawberries 19, 33, 41, 136, 137, 139, 140, 150
Stress xi, 43, 48, 57, 59, 60, 70, 72, 75, 77, 79, 80, 82, 83, 96, 97, 103, 165, 166, 169, 170, 171, 207, 216, 219, 222
Stroke 12, 19, 49, 78, 79, 83, 167
Sugar vi, 13, 14, 15, 16, 18, 21, 25, 27, 35, 40, 41, 48, 49, 51, 66, 77, 80, 82, 83, 85, 86, 89, 92, 93, 96, 103, 115, 116, 120, 123, 124, 130, 135, 138, 141, 144, 153, 155, 169, 170, 183, 185, 220
Sun 99, 100, 101, 174, 184, 207
Sunburns 174, 184
Sun exposure 99, 100, 101, 174, 184, 207
Sunscreen 100, 102
Sushi 38, 122, 145, 150, 158
Sweet potatoes 14, 26, 124, 125, 135
Sweets 85, 183
Swimming 16, 70
Swimming 72

T

Tendinitis 107
Testosterone 19, 79, 80, 218
Testosterone replacement 79, 218
Tilapia 39
TNF-alpha 68, 116
Tomatoes 124, 139
Tomatoes 25
Toro 38
Triglycerides 13, 63, 64, 77, 83, 123, 176
Tuna 22, 27, 37, 38, 111, 122, 148, 150
Turbinates 3, 201
Turkey 24, 25, 26, 27, 40, 50, 55, 111, 112, 113, 120, 121, 125, 129, 139, 140, 142,

147, 149, 187
Turkey burgers 55, 149
Turkey chili 50
Turkey meatballs 112, 113
Turkey meatballs 141
Turmeric 21, 25, 26, 29, 32, 57, 58, 60, 61, 62, 93, 108, 113, 135, 141, 143, 146, 148, 156, 159, 215, 223
Type 2 diabetes 12, 13, 14, 15, 16, 49, 86, 168, 219

U

UV radiation 60, 100

V

Vaccine ix, xv, xvi, 172
Vasomotor xviii, 4
Ventilator x, 69, 71
Ventilators 164
Vertebral disk disease 108
Vinegar 16, 23, 24, 26, 27, 42, 47, 48, 49, 89, 92, 93, 94, 111, 129, 130, 135, 137, 139, 140, 145, 146, 147, 149, 151, 153, 155, 157, 160, 161, 214
Visceral fat xi, 13, 71, 77, 78, 123, 165, 166, 170, 180, 206, 210, 218
Vitamin C 60, 66, 125, 168, 169, 179
Vitamin E 50, 60, 64, 66
Vitamin K 66
Vitamin K 52

W

Waistline vi, xvi, xvii, 12, 15, 16, 20, 74, 75, 77, 78, 79, 82, 83, 95, 153, 180, 181
Walking 16, 70, 72
Walnuts 22, 26, 87, 89, 139, 146, 149, 150
Water 3, 15, 19, 31, 35, 37, 39, 40, 42, 51, 55, 56, 64, 66, 91, 93, 94, 101, 102, 129, 130, 131, 132, 133, 134, 135, 137, 138, 139, 140, 141, 142, 143, 145, 146, 147, 148, 149, 150, 151, 155, 156, 157, 158, 159, 160, 161, 185, 213, 220
Weight gain 117, 170, 171
Weight loss xvii, 21, 43, 56, 81, 86, 91, 92, 93, 99, 100, 107, 109, 181
Weight training 69, 70
Weil 14, 113, 126
Wheat bread 134
Whey protein 20
White blood cells 9, 118
Wild salmon 36, 37, 89, 94
Wild salmon 36, 37
Wine 8, 56, 65, 81, 82, 102, 116, 117, 119, 129, 131, 133, 134, 138, 140, 185

Y

Yoga 74, 75, 218

NOTES

NOTES

NOTES

NOTES

FIGURE LEGEND

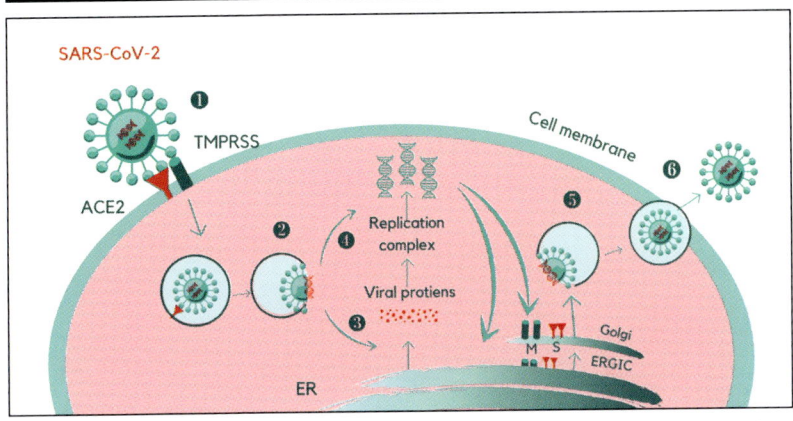

FIGURE 1. SARS-CoV-2 attaches to the receptor protein -- ACE2 -- and the TMPRSS2 protease in cells in different organs, including the cells on the inner lining of the nose. The mucus-producing goblet cells and ciliated cells in the nose had the highest levels of both these SARS-CoV-2 virus proteins, of all cells in the airways. This makes these cells the most likely initial infection route for the virus. [1] Spike protein on the virion binds to ACE2, a cell-surface protein. TMPRSS2, an enzyme, helps the virion enter [2] The virion releases its RNA [3] Some RNA is translated into proteins by the cell's machinery [4] Some of these proteins form a replication complex to make more RNA [5] Proteins and RNA are assembled into a new virion in the Golgi and [6] released. Sources: Song et al., 'Viruses', 2019; Jiang et al., 'Emerging Microbes and Infections, 2012; 'The Economist'.

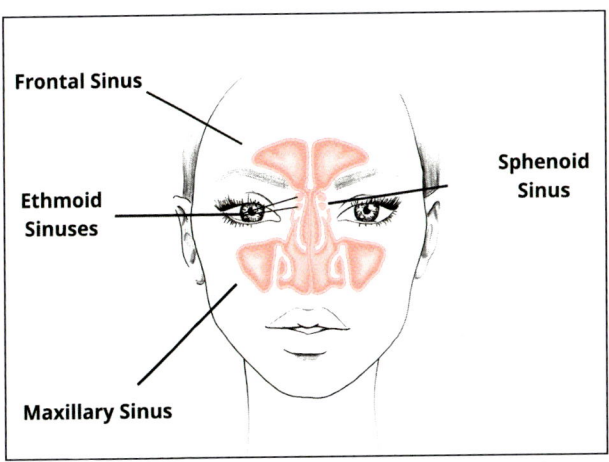

FIGURE 2. There are four sets of sinuses in your head. There are paired frontal, ethmoid, maxillary sinuses and a sphenoid sinus.

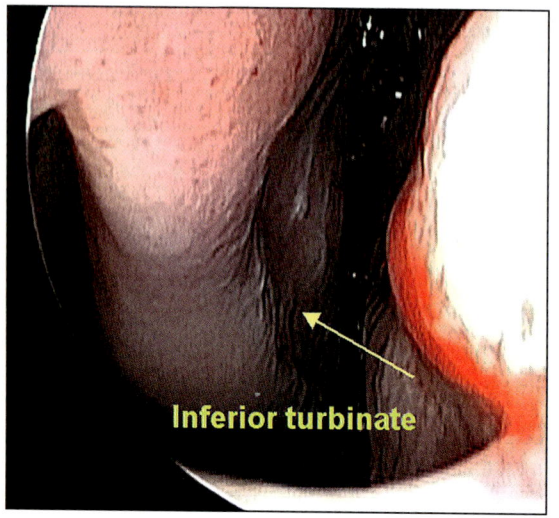

FIGURE 3. There are paired inferior turbinates in your nose that act to humidify the air that passes through the nasal passages.

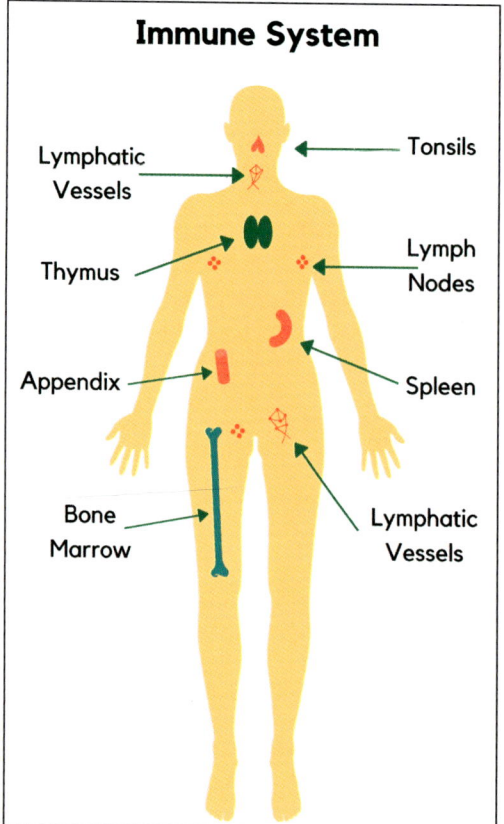

FIGURE 4. The organs of the immune system produce infection fighting cells and include your lymph nodes, lymphatic vessels as well as your bone marrow and other organs.

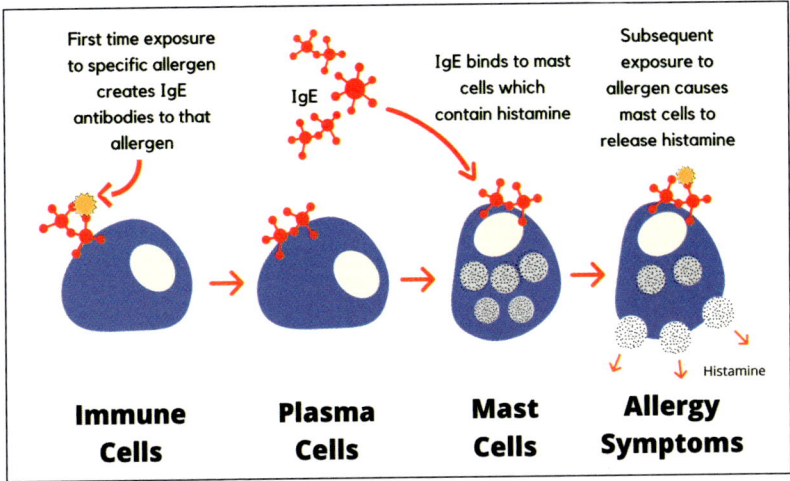

FIGURE 5. The role of antibodies and mast cells in allergy.

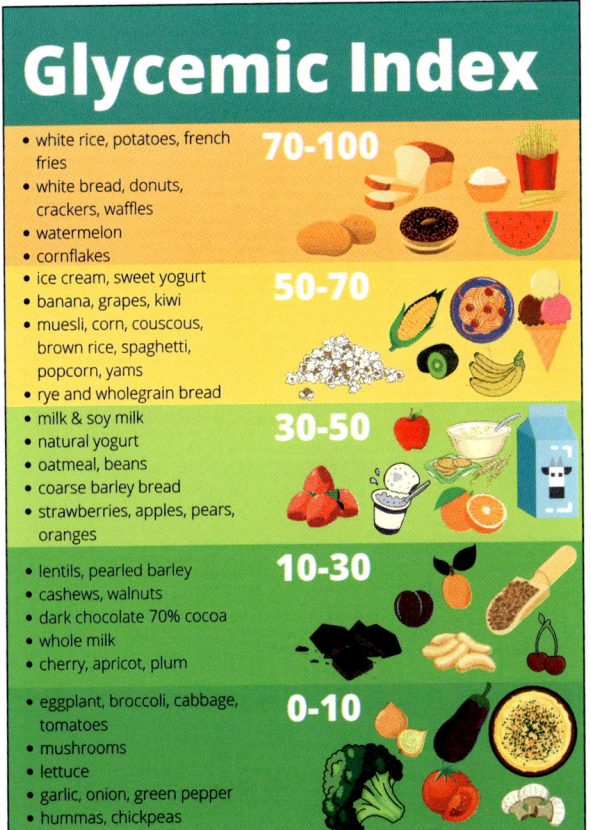

FIGURE 6. The glycemic index rates different foods on a scale from 0 to 100 representing the relative rise in blood glucose two hours after consuming that food.

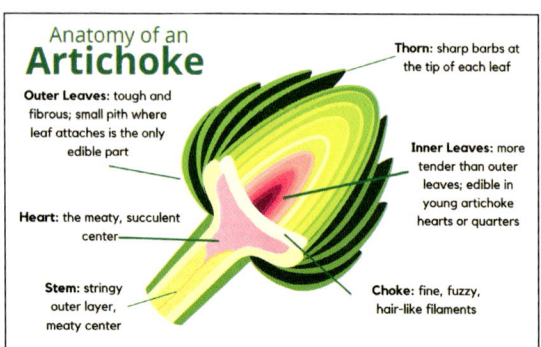

FIGURE 7. Anatomy of an artichoke.

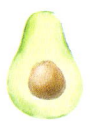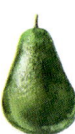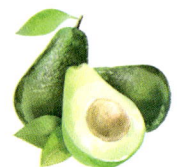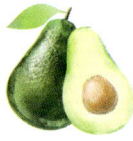

FIGURE 8. Benefits of avocado oil include a smoke point of 400 degrees F.

ANTI-INFLAMMATORY DIET IN THE ERA OF COVID-19 209

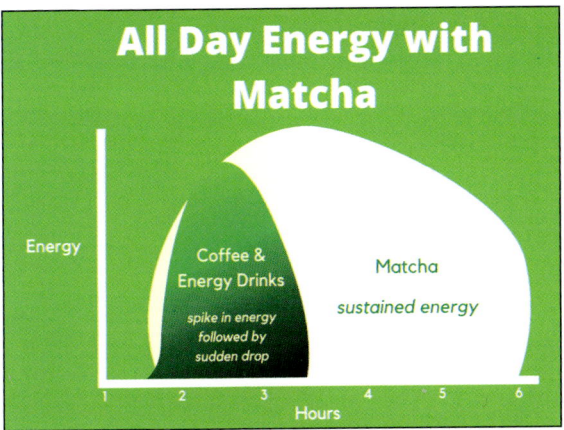

FIGURE 9. Matcha provides a prolonged caffeine effect without the spike in energy experienced with coffee and energy drinks.

BENEFITS OF MATCHA

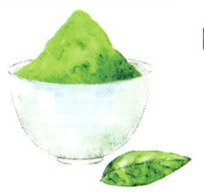

HEALTH BENEFITS

- Matcha contains L-Theanine, which is shown to increase focus and mental stamina
- High levels of anti-oxidents

CAFFIENE

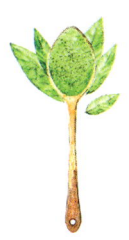

- A cup of matcha tea contains about 40 mg of caffeine
- Matcha has 50% less caffeine than coffee
- The energy from matcha is sustained for 4-6 hours with no jittery feeling or crash

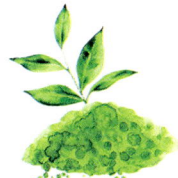

MATCHA PLANT

After green tea leaves are harvested and steamed, it goes through a process of drying. Once leaves are dried, it moves on to grinding through the stone mill which produces matcha powder.

FIGURE 10. Matcha has a higher level of anti-oxidants than most foods as well as many other health benefits.

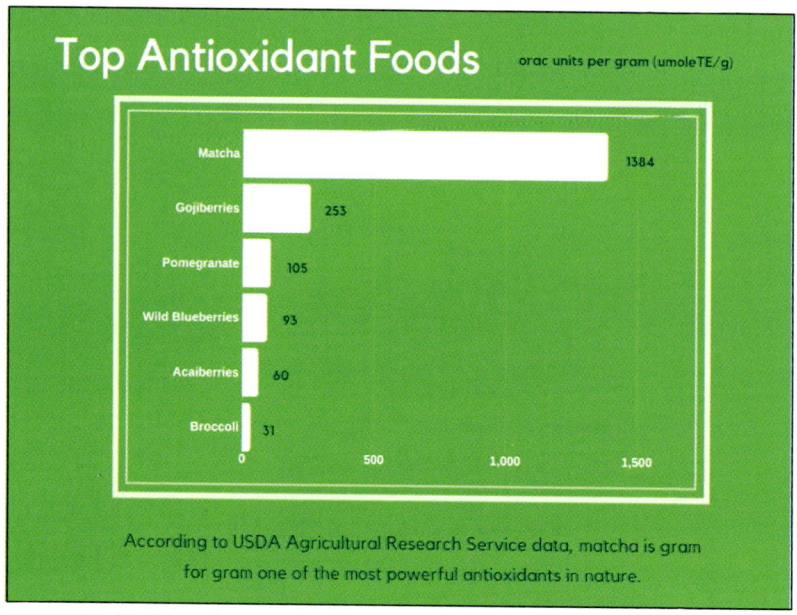

FIGURE 11. List of top antioxidants foods showing the very high levels in matcha.

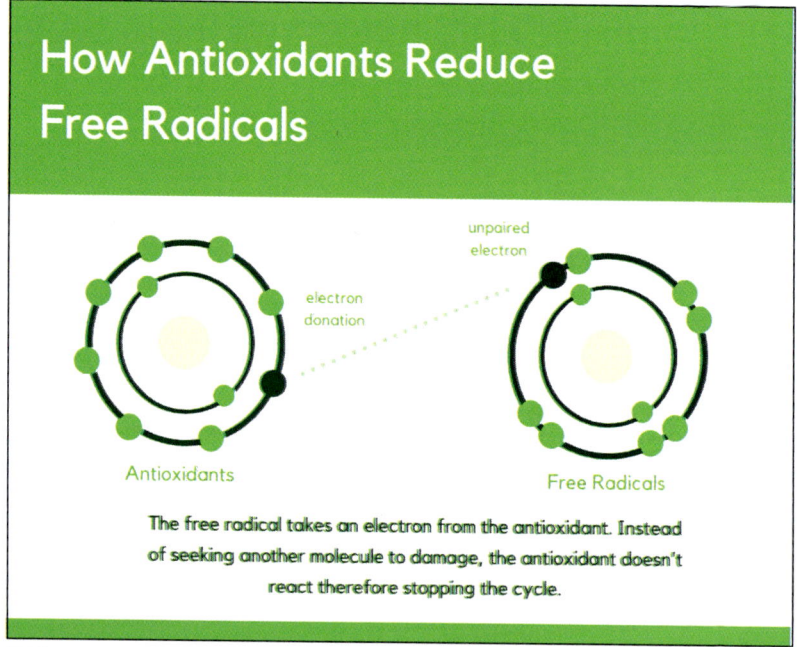

FIGURE 12. How antioxidants reduce free radicals.

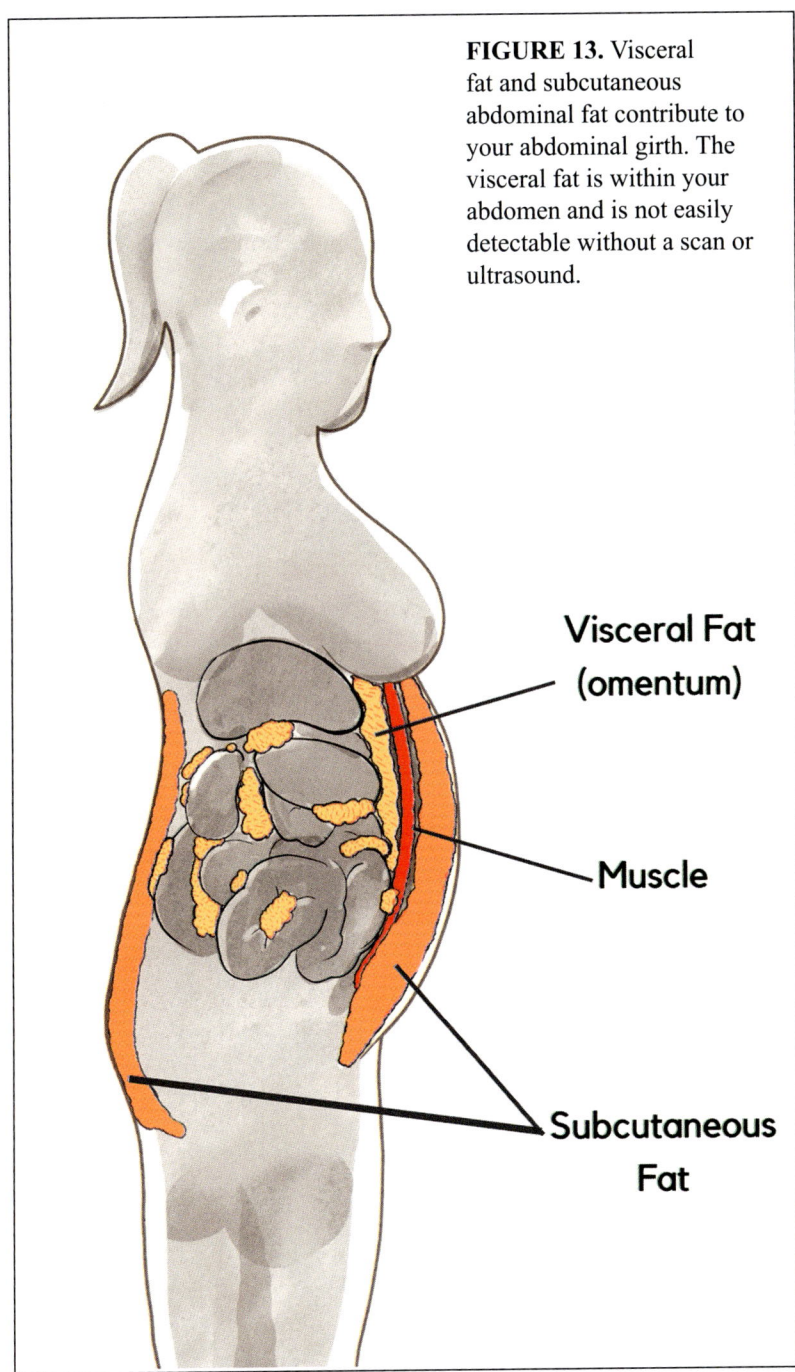

FIGURE 13. Visceral fat and subcutaneous abdominal fat contribute to your abdominal girth. The visceral fat is within your abdomen and is not easily detectable without a scan or ultrasound.

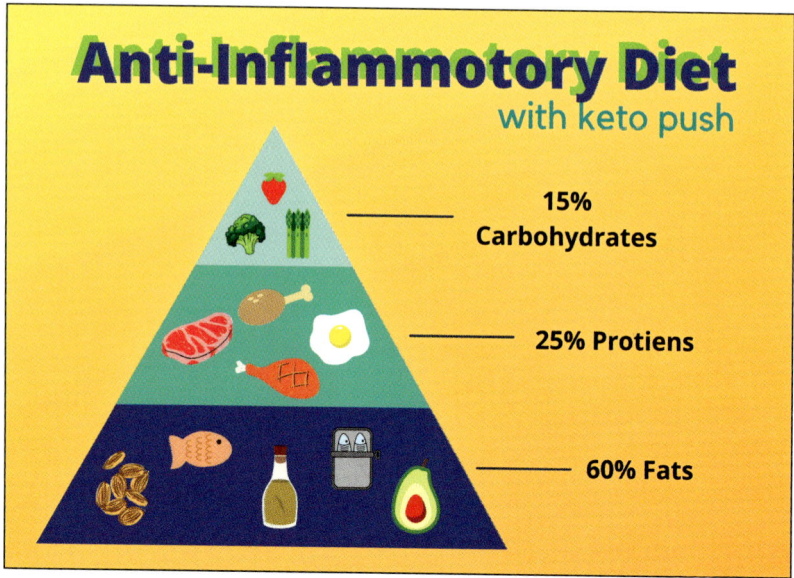

FIGURE 14. The anti-inflammatory diet with keto push (AI-keto diet) has a composition of 15% complex carbohydrates, 25% proteins and 60% healthy fats. This is different from the typical keto diet that is 5% to 10% carbs, 10% to 20% protein and 70% to 80% fat. The AI-keto diet differs in that the foods are anti-inflammatory in nature.

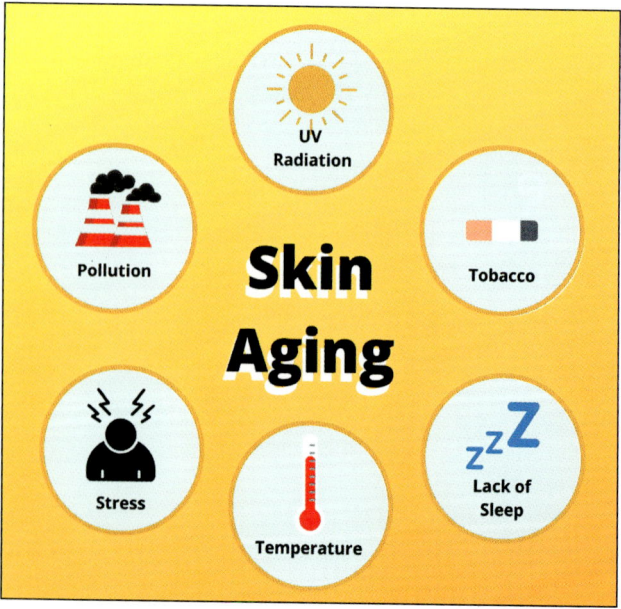

FIGURE 15. Aging of the skin can occur from sun exposure, tobacco use, stress as well as other factors.

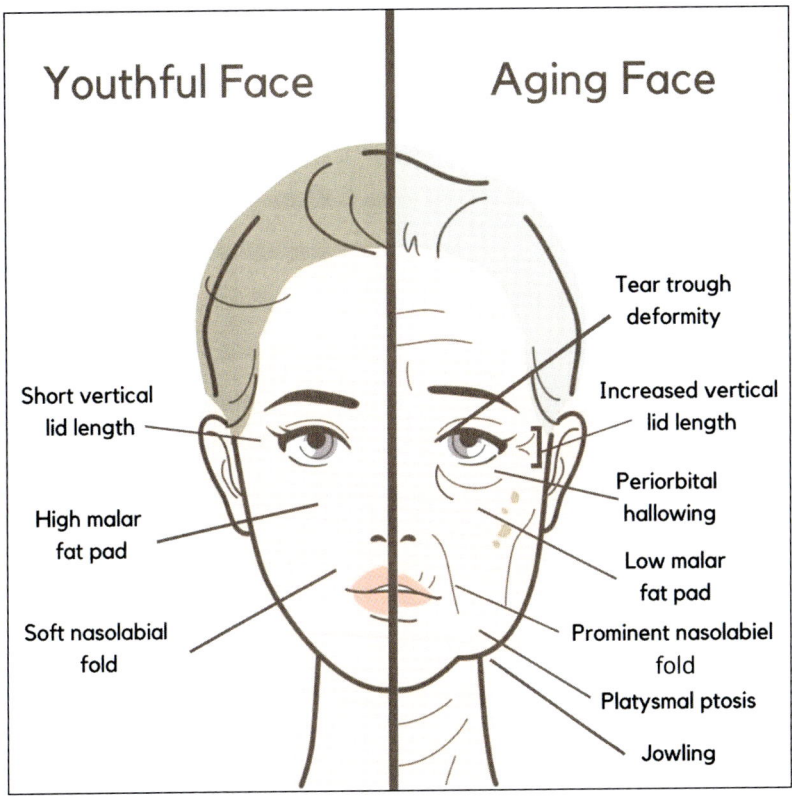

FIGURE 16. As you age, you will tend to lose fat in your face. With the loss of facial fat the skin tends to droop creating an aged look.

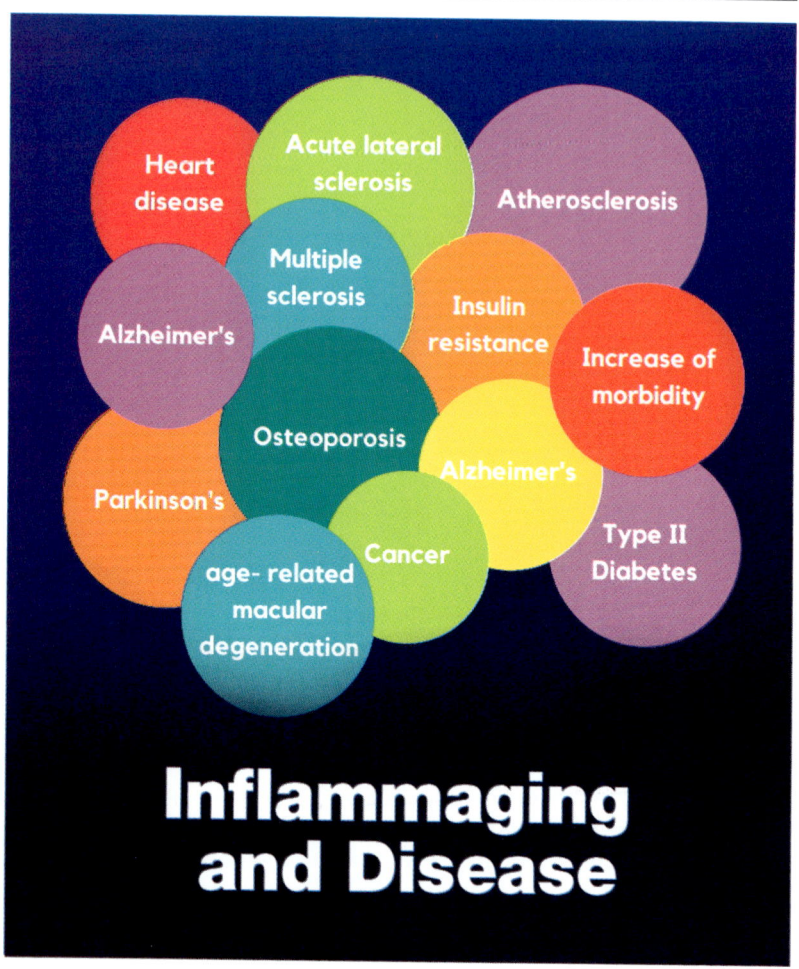

FIGURE 17. Inflammaging is a chronic low-grade inflammation that develops with advanced age and is believed to accelerate the process of biological aging and worsen many age-related diseases.

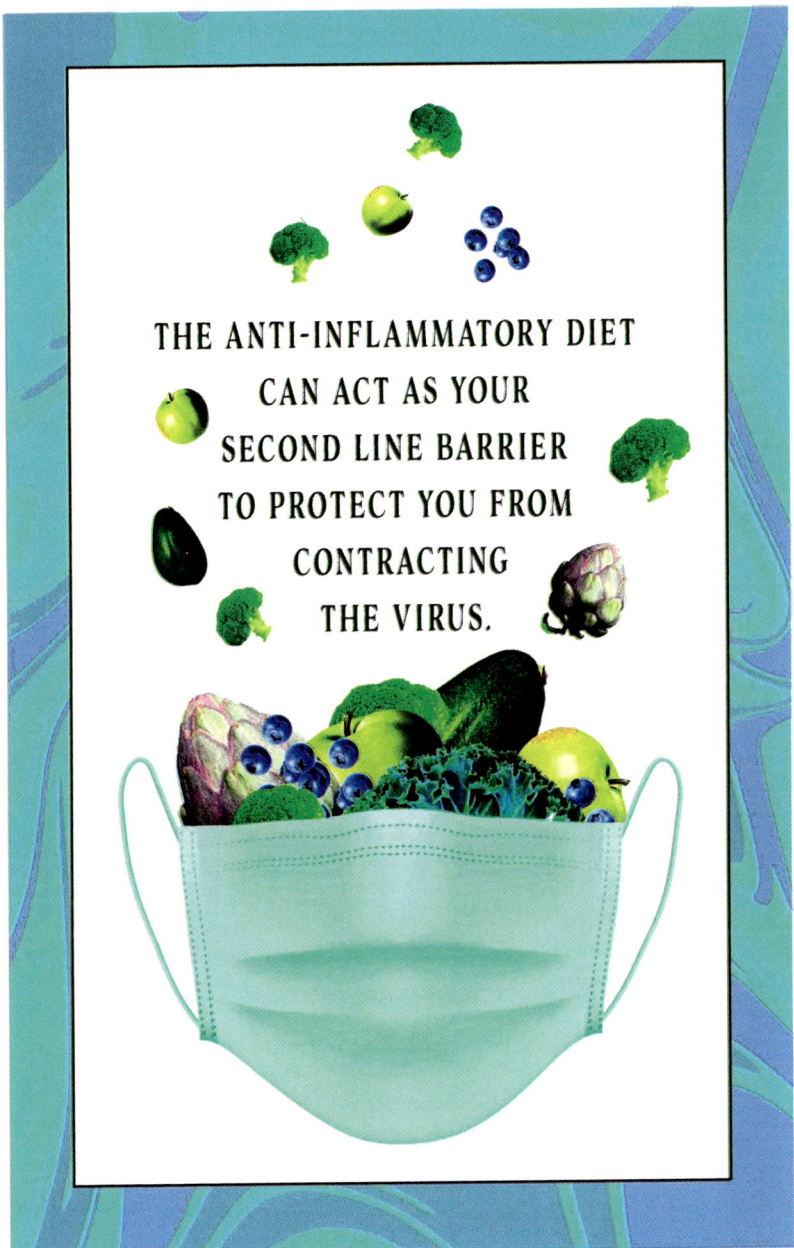

FIGURE 18. In addition to wearing a mask and social distancing, the anti-inflammatory diet can act as another barrier to protect you from contracting Covid-19.

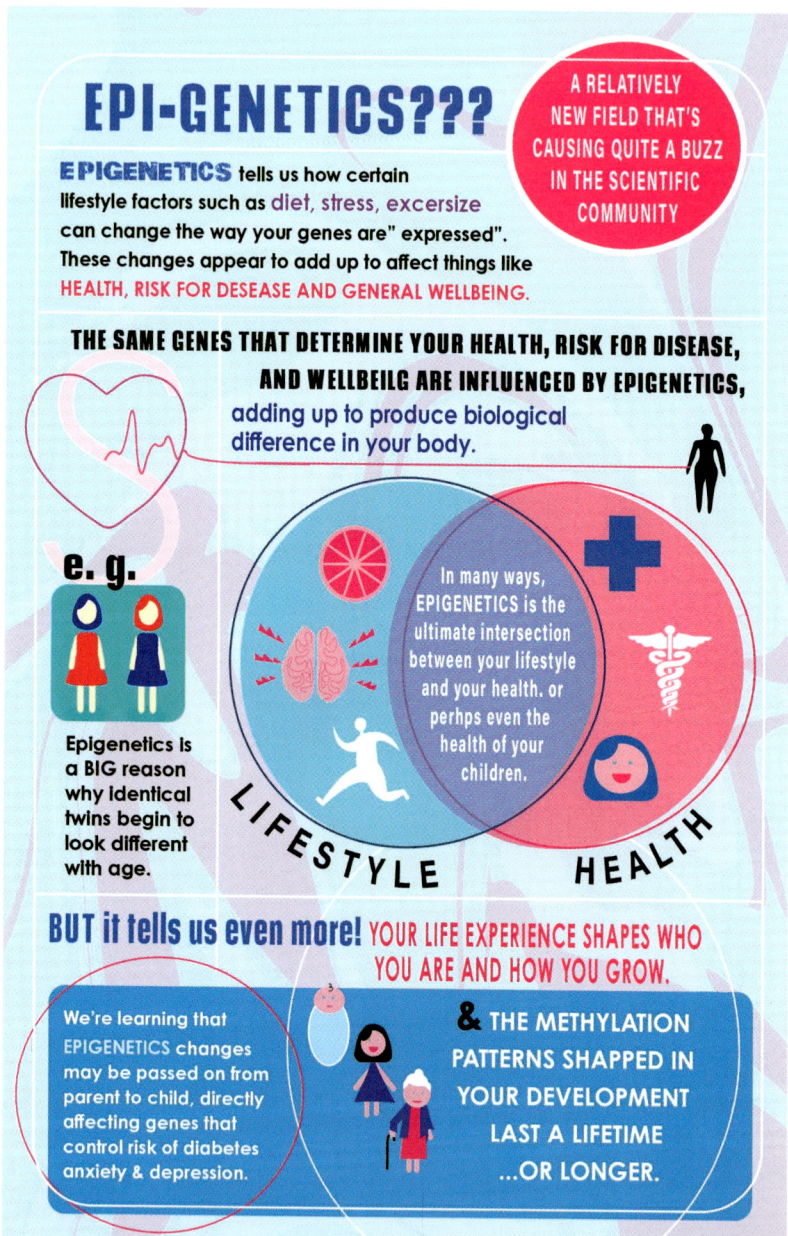

FIGURE 19. Epigenetics is a new area of study that shows how genes can be turned on or off based on your lifestyle choices. The effects can impact your children and grandchildren.

NATIONAL COVID-19 AND MENTAL HEALTH STUDY
BASED ON A NATIONAL SURVEY, WITH 4,149 RESPONDENTS

61% Feeling more stress.

60% Feeling more nervous, anxious or on edge.

39% Eating more than normal.

61% Having same amount of sex with partner

47% Feeling trapped at home

54% Feeling very concerned about catching Covid 19.

69% Distracting themselves with activities.

48% Looked for some good in what is happening.

FIGURE 20. Chapman mental health study. Taken from the Chapman University National Covid-19 and mental health study. April 2020.

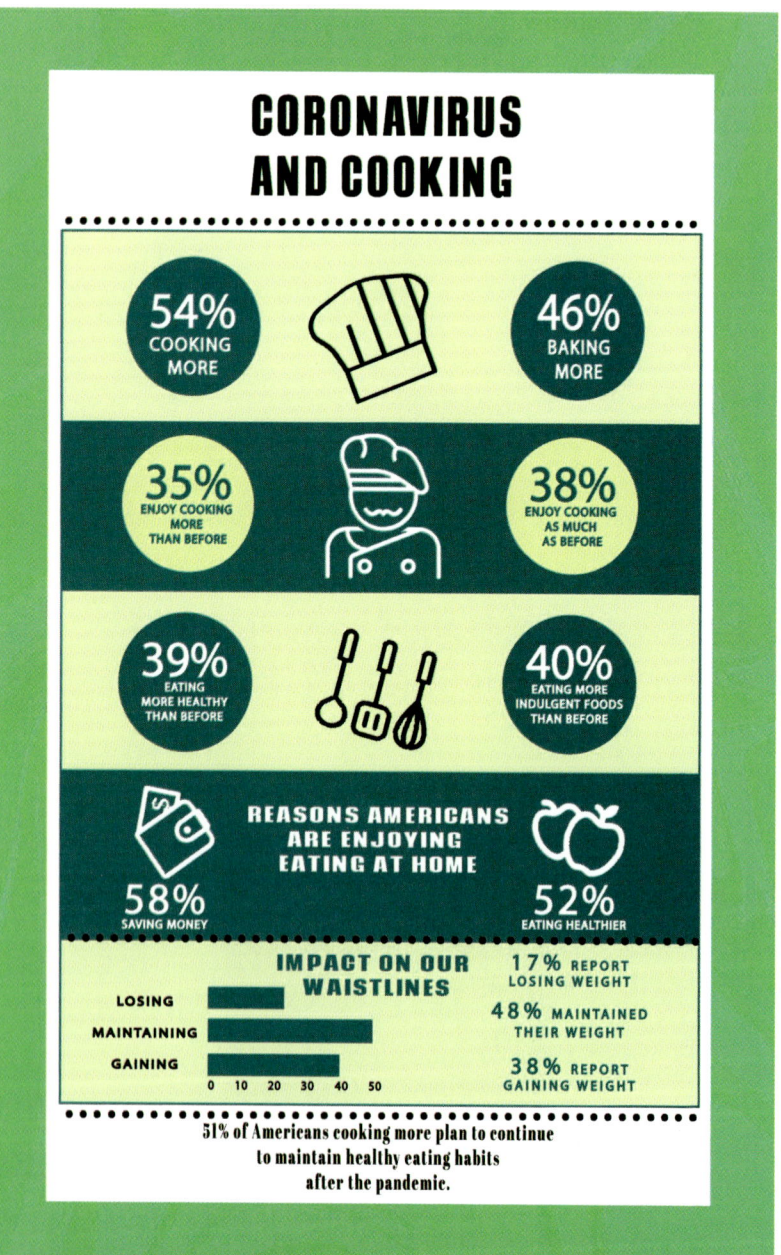

FIGURE 21. More people started to cook during the pandemic with a focus on eating healthier. From Hunter Food Study, April 2020.

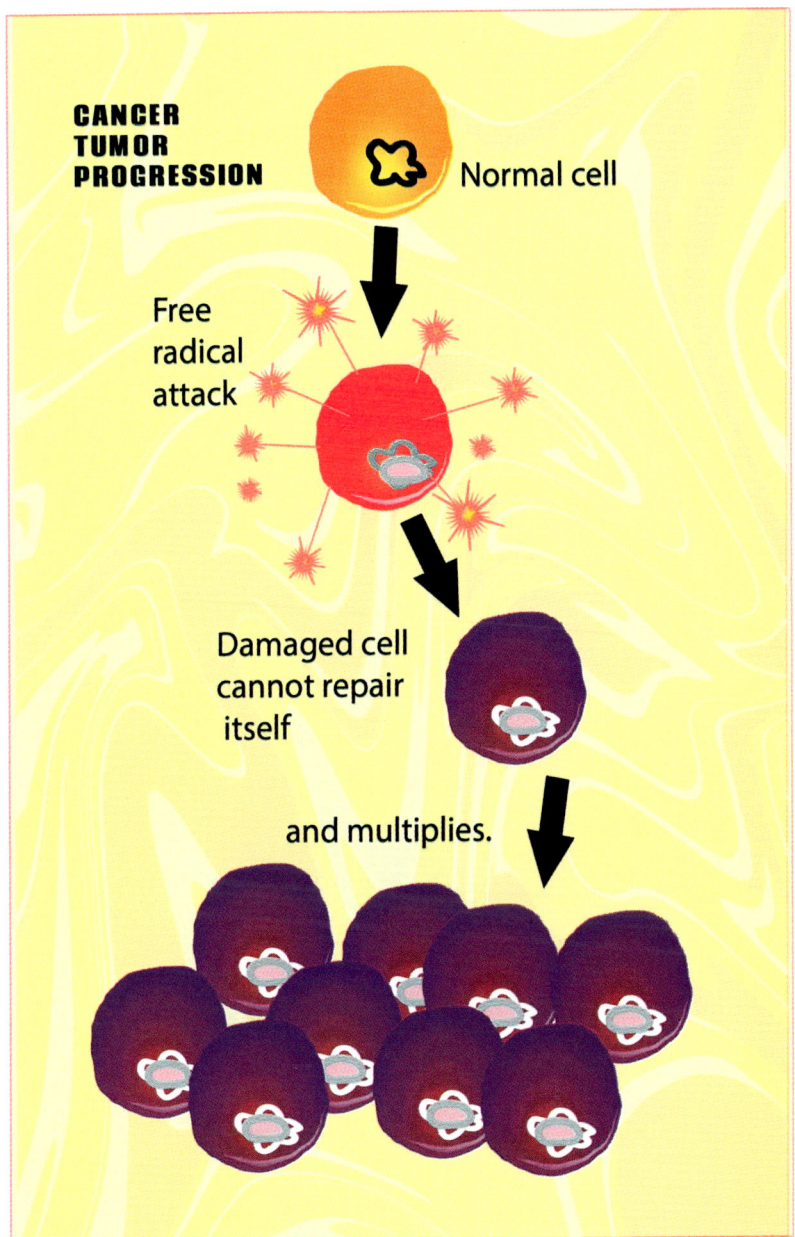

FIGURE 22. Skin cancer can form from sun exposure and other environmental factors that form free radicals that attack cells resulting in cancer cells.

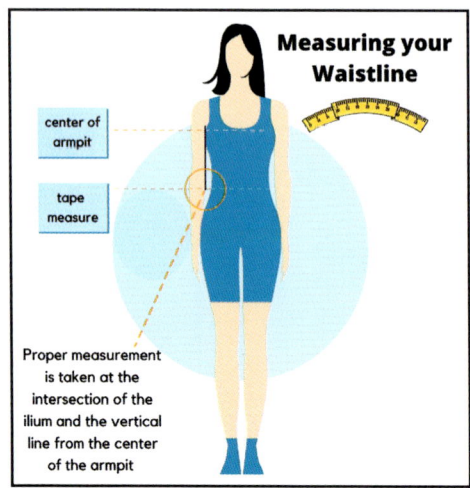

FIGURE 23. Method of measuring your waistline.

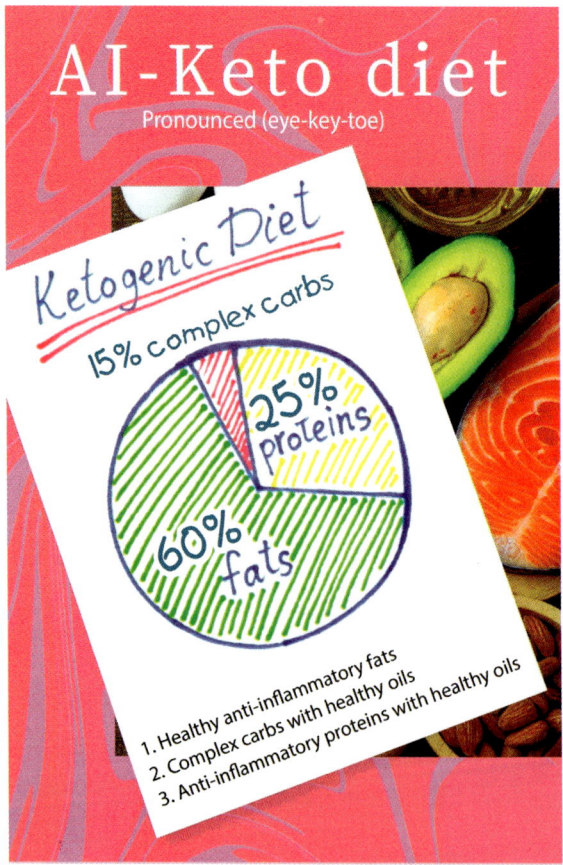

FIGURE 24. The AI-keto diet is a combination of the anti-inflammatory diet and the ketogenic diet.

References

1 Wortham JM. et al. Characteristics of persons who died with COVID-19 — United States, February 12–May 18, 2020. Morbidity and Mortality Weekly Report (MMWR) Jul 17, 2020; 69(28):923-929.

2 Chowdhury MA. Immune response in COVID-19: A review. Journal of Infection and Public Health. https://doi.org/10.1016/j.jiph.2020.07.001.

3 Sanyaolu A, et al. Comorbidity and its impact on patients with COVID-19. SN Compr Clin Med. Jun 25 2020:1–8.

doi: 10.1007/s42399-020-00363-4.

4 Butler MJ, Barrientos RM. The impact of nutrition on COVID-19 susceptibility and long-term consequences. Brain Behav Immun. Jul 2020;87:53–54. Published online 2020 Apr 18. doi: 10.1016/j.bbi.2020.04.040

5 Zabetakis I. COVID-19: The inflammation link and the role of nutrition in potential mitigation. Nutrients. May 2020;12(5):1466. Published online 2020 May 19. doi: 10.3390/nu12051466.

6 Nam SY, et al. The effect of abdominal visceral fat, circulating inflammatory cytokines, and leptin levels on reflux esophagitis. J Neurogastroenterol Motil. 2015;21(2): 247-254 https://doi.org/10.5056/jnm14114.

7 Yang J, Zheng Y, Gou X, Pu K, Chen Z, Guo Q, Ji R, Wang H, Wang Y, Zhou Y. Prevalence of comorbidities and its effects in coronavirus disease 2019 patients: a systematic review and meta-analysis. Int J Infect Dis. Mar 2020; 12(94):91-95.

8 Galea et al. The mental health consequences of Covid-19 and physical distancing. JAMA Intern Med. 2020;180(6):817-818. doi:10.1001/jamainternmed.2020.1562.

9 Cauley et al. Direct costs of adult chronic rhinosinusitis by using 4 methods of estimation: Results of the US medical expenditure panel survey. Rhinitis, sinusitis, and upper airway disease. Dec 1, 2015;136(6):1517-1522.

10 Sungnak et al. SAR-CoV-2 entry factors are highly expressed in nasal epithelial cells together with innate genes. Nature Medicine. Apr 23, 2020.

11 Speth et al. Olfactory dysfunction and sinonasal symptomatology in Covid-19: 2prevalence, severity, timing and associated characteristics. Otolaryngology-Head&NeckSurgery.

12 Yan C, Faraji F, Prajapati DP, Boone CE, DeConde AS. Association of chemosensory dysfunction and Covid 19 in patients presenting with influenza like symptoms. https://doi.org/10.1002/alr.22579.

13 Suzuki M, Saito K, Min W-P, et al. Identification of viruses in patients with postviral olfactory dysfunction: The Laryngoscope. 2007;117(2):272-277.

14 Brann D, Tsukahara T, Weinreb C, Logan DW, Datta SR. Non-neural expression of SARS-CoV-2 entry genes in the olfactory epithelium suggests mechanisms underlying anosmia in Covid-19 patients. Neuroscience. 2020.

15 Galli SJ. The development of allergic inflammation. Nature. Jul 24, 2008; 454(7203): 445–454.

16 Kawasaki E. Type 1 Diabetes and autoimmunity. Clin Pediatr Endocrinol. Oct 2014;23(4):99–105.

17 Sacks Frank M, Carey Vincent J, Anderson Cheryl A M, et al. Effects of high vs low glycemic index of dietary carbohydrate on cardiovascular disease risk factors and insulin sensitivity: the omniCarb randomized clinical trial. JAMA. Dec 17, 2014;312(23):2531-2541

18 Sangal N, Sangal A. Dietary carbohydrates and glycemic index: a systematic review. In: Flaps PD, ed. New Developments in Nutrition Research. New York: Nova Science Publishers; 2006:99-115.

19 Mohammadi□Sartang et al. The effect of flaxseed supplementation on body weight and body composition: a systematic review and meta□analysis of 45 randomized placebo□controlled trials. Obesity Reviews. Sep 2017;18(9):1096-1107.

20 Salas-Salvador et al. Effect of two doses of a mixture of soluble fibres on body weight and metabolic variables in overweight or obese patients: a randomised tTrial. Br J Nutr. Jun 2008;99(6):1380-7.

21 Barnett JR. The science of soy: what do we really know? Environ Health Perspect. Jul 2006;114(6):A352–A358.

22 Schäfer G, Kaschula CH. The immunomodulation and anti-Inflammatory effects of garlic organosulfur compounds in cancer chemoprevention. Anticancer Agents Med Chem. Feb 2014;14(2): 233–240.

23 Varshney R, Budoff MJ. Garlic and heart disease. J Nutr. Feb 2016;146(2):416S-421S. doi: 10.3945/jn.114.202333. Epub 2016 Jan 13.

24 Burton P, Lightowler HJ. The impact of freezing and toasting on the glycaemic response of white bread. Eur J Clin Nutr. May 2008;62(5):594-9. Epub 2007 Apr 4.

25 J Agric Food Chem. Dec 27,2006;54(26):9966-77.

26 Johnson Jodee L., Gonzalez de Mejia Elvira. Flavonoid apigenin modified gene expression associated with inflammation and cancer and induced apoptosis in human pancreatic cancer cells through inhibition of GSK-3β/NF-κB signaling cascade. Molecular Nutrition & Food Research. 2013;doi: 10.1002/mnfr.201300307.

27 J Altern. Artichoke leaf extract reduces symptoms of irritable bowel syndrome and improves quality of life in otherwise healthy volunteers suffering from concomitant dyspepsia: a subset analysis.Complement Med. Aug 2004;10(4):667-9.

28 Baranski M. et al. Higher antioxidant and lower cadmium concentrations and lower incidence of pesticide residues in organically grown crops: a systematic literature review and meta-analyses.Br J Nutr. Sep 2014 14;112(5):794-811. doi: 10.1017/S0007114514001366. Epub 2014 Jun 26.

29 Vandenberg et al. Is it time to reassess current safety standards for glyphosate-based herbicides? Vandenberg LN, et al. J Epidemiol Community Health. 2017;71:613–618. doi:10.1136/jech-2016-208463.

30 Fritsche KL. The science of fatty acids and inflammation. Adv Nutr. May 2015;6(3):293S–301S.

31 Van Elswyk, McNeill SH. Impact of grass/forage feeding versus grain finishing on beef nutrients and sensory quality: the U.S. experience. Meat Sci. Jan 2014;96(1):535-40.

32 Reinagel Monica with Julius Torelli, M.D. The Inflammation-Free Diet Plan: The Scientific Way to Lose Weight, Banish Pain, Prevent Disease, and Slow Aging. McGraw-Hill; 2006.

33 McCarty MF, DiNicolantonio JJ, O'Keefe JH. Capsaicin may have important potential for promoting vascular and metabolic health. Open Heart. Jun 17, 2015;2(1):e000262.

34 Dailey et al. The microbiota of freshwater fish and freshwater niches contain omega-3 fatty acid-producing shewanella species. Appl Environ Microbiol. Jan 1, 2016;82(1):218–231.

35 Wu SH, Shu XO, Chow WH, et al. Soy food intake and circulating levels of inflammatory markers in Chinese women. J Acad Nutr Diet. 2012;112:996-1004.

36 Giuliana Noratto et al. Assessing non-digestible compounds in apple cultivars and their potential as modulators of obese faecal microbiota in vitro. Food Chemistry. doi: 10.1016/j.foodchem.2014.03.122.

37 Gray B, Steyn F, Davies PS, Vitetta L. Omega-3 fatty acids: a review of the effects on adiponectin and leptin and potential implications for obesity management. Eur J Clin Nutr. 2013 Dec;67(12):1234-42.

38 Evero N, Hackett LC, Clark RD, Phelan S, Hagobian TA. Aerobic exercise reduces neuronal responses in food reward brain regions. J Appl Physiol (1985). May 2012;112(9):1612-9.

39 Schubert MM, Sabapathy S, Leveritt M, Desbrow B. Acute exercise and hormones related to appetite regulation: a meta-analysis. Sports Med. Mar 2014;44(3):387-403.

40 Forde CG, van Kuijk N, Thaler T, de Graaf C, Martin N. Oral processing characteristics of solid savoury meal components, and relationship with food composition, sensory attributes and expected satiation. Appetite. Jan 2013;60(1):208-219.

41 Corney RA, Sunderland C, James LJ. Immediate pre-meal water ingestion decreases voluntary food intake in lean young males. Eur J Nutr. Mar 2016;55(2):815-819.

42 Groesz L, McCoy S, Carl J, Saslow L, Stewart J, Adler N, Laraia B, and Epel E. What is eating you? Stress and the Drive to Eat. Appetite. Apr 2012;58(2):717–721.

43 Cicerale S., Lucas L.J., Keast R.S. Antimicrobial, antioxidant and anti-inflammatory phenolic activities in extra-virginextra-virgin olive oil. Curr. Opin. Biotechnol. 2012;23:129–135.

44 (Beauchamp, G.K., Keast, R.S.J., Morel, D., Lin, J.,Pika, J., Han, Q., Lee, C-H, Smith, A.B. III, Breslin, P.A.S.Ibuprofen-like activity in extra-virgin olive oil. Nature. 2005;437:45-6.

45 Karkoula E, Skantzari A, Melliou E, Magiatis P. Quantitative measurement of major secoiridoid derivatives in olive oil using qNMR. Proof of the artificial formation of aldehydic oleuropein and ligstroside aglycon isomers. J Agric Food Chem. Jan 22, 2014;62(3):600-7.

46 Keys A. Coronary heart disease in seven countries. Circulation. 1970;41:186–195.

47 WHO. World Health Statistics 2010. World Health Organization; Geneva, Switzerland: 2010.

48 Corona G., Spencer J., Dessi M. Extra-virgin olive oil phenolics: Absorption, metabolism, and biological activities in the GI tract. Toxicol. Ind. Health. 2009;25:285–293.

49 Peyrot des Gachons C., Uchida K., Bryant B., Shima A., Sperry J.B., Dankulich-Nagrudny L., Tominaga M., Smith A.B., 3rd, Beauchamp G.K., Breslin P.A. Unusual pungency from extra-virgin olive oil is attributable to restricted spatial expression of the receptor of oleocanthal. J. Neurosci. 2011;31:999–1009. doi: 10.1523/JNEUROSCI.1374-10.2011.

50 Karkoula E., Skantzari A., Melliou E., Magiatis P. Direct measurement of oleocanthal and oleacein levels in olive oil by quantitative 1H-NMR. Establishment of a new index for the characterization of extra-virgin olive oils. J. Agric. Food Chem. 2012;60:11696–11703.

51 Beauchamp G.K., Keast R.S., Morel D., Lin J., Pika J., Han Q., Lee C.H., Smith A.B., Breslin P.A. Phytochemistry: Ibuprofen-like activity in extra-virgin olive oil. Nature. 2005;437:45–46. doi: 10.1038/437045a.

52 Gonzalez C.A., Riboli E. Diet and cancer prevention: contributions from the European Prospective Investigation into Cancer and Nutrition (EPIC) study. Eur. J. Cancer. 2010;46:2555–2562.

53 De Lorgeril M., Salen P., Martin J.-L., Monjaud I., Boucher P., Mamelle N. Mediterranean dietary pattern in a randomized trial: Prolonged survival and possible reduced cancer rate. Arch. Intern. Med. 1998;158:1181–1187. doi: 10.1001/archinte.158.11.1181.

54 Scotece M., Gómez R., Conde J., Lopez V., Gómez-Reino J.J., Lago F., Smith A.B., Gualillo O. Further evidence for the anti-inflammatory activity of oleocanthal: inhibition of MIP-1α and IL-6 in J774 macrophages and in ATDC5 chondrocytes. Life Sci. 2012;91:1229–1235.

55 Monti M.C., Margarucci L., Tosco A., Riccio R., Casapullo A. New insights on the interaction mechanism between tau protein and oleocanthal, an extra-virgin olive-oil bioactive component. Food Funct. 2011;2:423–428.

56 Pitt J., Roth W., Lacor P., Blankenship M., Velasco P., de Felice F., Breslin P.A., Klein W.L. Alzheimer's-associated A-beta oligomers show altered structure, immunoreactivity and synaptic toxicity with low doses of oleocanthal. Toxicol. Appl. Pharmacol. 2009;240:189–197.

57 Scarmeas N., Luchsinger J.A., Schupf N., Brickman A.M., Cosentino S., Tang M.X., Stern Y. Physical activity, diet, and risk of Alzheimer disease. J. Am. Med. Assoc. 2009;302:627–637.

58 Scalbert A, Manach C, Morand C, Remesy C, Jimenez L. Dietary polyphenols and the prevention of diseases. Crit Rev Food Sci Nutr. 2005;45:287–306.

59 Carol S. Johnston, PhD, RD and Cindy A. Gaas, BS The grapes that are used to make balsamic vinegar contain antioxidants that fight against cell damage, improve the body's immune system. Vinegar: medicinal uses and antiglycemic effect. Med Gen Med. 2006;8(2):61.

60 Chatterjee S, Jungraithmayr W, Bagchi D. Immunity and inflammation in health and disease emerging roles of nutraceuticals and functional foods in immune support. ScienceDirect. 2017.

61 Bazina N, He J. Analysis of fatty acid profiles of free fatty acids generated in deep-frying process. J Food Sci Technol. Aug 2018;55(8):3085-3092. doi: 10.1007/s13197-018-3232-9. Epub 2018 May 16.

62 Gray S. Cooking with Extra-virgin olive oil. ACNEM Journal Vol 34 No 2 ,2015.

63 Flores Marcos et al. Avocado oil: characteristics, properties, and applications. Molecules. 2019 Jun; 24(11): 2172.

64 Hsu E, Parthasarathy S. Anti-inflammatory and antioxidant effects of sesame oil on atherosclerosis: a descriptive literature review. Cureus. Jul 2017;9(7):e1438.

65 Babu, P.V.; Liu, D. Green tea catechins and cardiovascular health: An update. Curr. Med. Chem. 2008;15:1840–1850.

66 Henning, S.M.; Niu, Y.; Lee, N.H.; Thames, G.D.; Minutti, R.R.; Wang, H.; Go, V.L.; Heber, D. Bioavailability and antioxidant activity of tea flavonoids after consumption of green tea, black tea, or a green tea extract supplement. Am. J. Clin. Nutr. 2004;80:1558–1564.

67 Ju, J.; Lu, G.; Lambert, J.D.; Yang, C.S. Inhibition of carcinogenesis by tea constituents. Semin. Cancer Biol. 2007; 17:395–402.

68 Yang, C.S. Antioxidant and anti-carcinogenic activities of tea polyphenols. Arch. Toxicol. 2009;83:11–21.

69 Chainani-Wu N, Safety and Anti-Inflammatory Activity of Curcumin: A Component of Tumeric (Curcuma Longa).J Altern Complement Med Feb 2003;9(1):161-8.

70 Mashhadi NS. Anti-oxidative and anti-inflammatory effects of ginger in health and physical activity: review of current evidence. Int J Prev Med. Apr 2013;4(Suppl 1): S36–S42.

71 Aneja R. et al. Theaflavin, a black tea extract, is a novel anti-inflammatory compound. Crit Care Med. Oct 2004;32(10):2097-103.

72 Chatterjee P. et al. Evaluation of anti-inflammatory effects of green tea and black tea: A comparative in vitro study. J Adv Pharm Technol Res. Apr-Jun2012; (2):136–138.

73 Thring TSA. et al. Antioxidant and potential anti-inflammatory activity of extracts and formulations of white tea, rose, and witch hazel on primary human dermal fibroblast cells are reported. J Inflamm (Lond). 2011;8:27.

74 Srivastava JK. Chamomile, a novel and selective COX-2 inhibitor with anti-inflammatory activity. Life Sci. Nov 4, 2009;85(19-20):663–669.

75 Hewlings SW, Douglas S. Kalman DS. Curcumin: a review of its effects on human health. Foods. Oct 2017; 6(10): 92.

76 Menon VP, Sudheer AR. Antioxidant and anti-inflammatory properties of curcumin. Adv Exp Med Biol. 2007;595:105-25[Ma11].

77 Tayyem RF, Heath DD, Al-Delaimy WK, Rock CL. Curcumin content of turmeric and curry powders. Nutr Cancer. 2006;55(2):126-31.

78 Shoba G, Joy D, Joseph T, Majeed M, Rajendran R, Srinivas PS. Influence of piperine on the pharmacokinetics of curcumin in animals and human volunteers. Planta Med. May 1998;64(4):353-6.

79 Huang TL. Omega-3 fatty acids, cognitive decline, and Alzheimer's disease: a critical review and evaluation of the literature. J Alzheimers Dis. 2010;21(3):673-90. doi: 10.3233/JAD-2010-090934.

80 Calder PC. n-3 polyunsaturated fatty acids, inflammation, and inflammatory diseases. Am J Clin Nutr. Jun 2006;83(6 Suppl):1505S-1519S. doi: 10.1093/ajcn/83.6.1505S.

81 Federation of American Societies for Experimental Biology. Anti-inflammatory effects of omega-3 fatty acid In fish oil linked To lowering Of prostaglandin. Science Daily, 4 April 2006.

82 Kris-Etherton PM, Harris WS, Appel LJ. Omega-3 fatty acids and cardiovascular disease: new recommendations from the American Heart Association. Arterioscler Thromb Vasc Biol. Feb 1,2003;23(2):151-2.

83 Byelashov O, Sinclair A, Kaur G. Dietary sources, current intakes, and nutritional role of omega-3 docosapentaenoic acid. Lipid Technol. Apr 2015;27(4):79–82.

84 Neubronner J, Schuchardt JP, Kressel G, Merkel M, von Schacky C, Hahn A. Enhanced increase of omega-3 index in response to long-term n-3 fatty acid supplementation from triacylglycerides versus ethyl esters. Eur J Clin Nutr. Feb 2011;65(2):247-54. doi: 10.1038/ejcn.2010.239. Epub 2010 Nov 10.

85 Gerster, Helga. Can adults adequately convert a-linolenic acid (18: 3n-3) to eicosapentaenoic acid (20: 5n-3) and docosahexaenoic acid (22: 6n-3)? International Journal for Vitamin and Nutrition Research. 1998;68.3:159-173.

86 Riccioni G, Gammone MA, Tettamanti G, Bergante S, Pluchinotta FR, D'Orazio N. Resveratrol and anti-atherogenic effects. Int J Food Sci Nutr. 2015;66(6):603-10. doi: 10.3109/09637486.2015.1077796. Epub 2015 Aug 26.

87 Samsami-Kor M, Daryani NE, Asl PR, Hekmatdoost A. Anti-Inflammatory Effects of Resveratrol in Patients with Ulcerative Colitis: A Randomized, Double-Blind, Placebo-controlled Pilot Study. Arch Med Res. May 2015;46(4):280-5. doi: 10.1016/j.arcmed.2015.05.005. Epub 2015 May 20.

88 Colombo E, Sangiovanni E, Dell'agli M. A review on the anti-inflammatory activity of pomegranate in the gastrointestinal tract. Evid Based Complement Alternat Med. 2013;2013:247145. doi: 10.1155/2013/247145. Epub 2013 Mar 14.

89 Balbir-Gurman A, Fuhrman B, Braun-Moscovici Y, Markovits D, Aviram M. Consumption of pomegranate decreases serum oxidative stress and reduces disease activity in patients with active rheumatoid arthritis: a pilot study. Isr Med Assoc J. 2011 Aug;13(8):474-9.

90 Paller CJ, Pantuck A, Carducci, MA. A review of pomegranate in prostate cancer. Prostate Cancer Prostatic Dis. Sep 2017;20(3):265–270.

91 Sahebkar et al. Effects of pomegranate juice on blood pressure: a systematic review and meta-analysis of randomized controlled trials. Pharmacological Research. January 2017;115:149-1610.

92 Woods JA. The Covid-19 pandemic and physical activity. Sports Medicine and Health Science Available online 30 May 2020.

93 Bruunsgaard H, Pedersen BK. Age-related inflammatory cytokines and disease. Immunol Allergy Clin North Am. 2003;23:15–39.

94 Seshadri P, Iqbal N, Stern L, Williams M, Chicano KL, Daily DA, McGrory J, Gracely EJ, Rader DJ, Samaha FF. A randomized study comparing the effects of a low-carbohydrate diet and a conventional diet on lipoprotein subfractions and C-re-

active protein levels in patients with severe obesity. Am J Med. 2004;117:398–405.

95 Petersen AM, Pedersen BK. The anti-inflammatory effect of exercise. J Appl Physiol (1985). Apr 2005;98(4):1154-62.

96 Fuster JJ, Walsh K. The good, the bad, and the ugly of interleukin-6 signaling. EMBO J. Jul 1, 2014;33(13):1425–1427.

97 Pedersen BK. Anti inflammatory effects of exercise: role in diabetes and cardiovascular disease. 2017;47(8):600-611.

98 Dimitrova S, Hultenga E, Hong S. Inflammation and exercise: inhibition of monocytic intracellular TNF production by acute exercise via β2-adrenergic activation. Brain, Behavior, and Immunity. 2017;61:60-68.

99 Yan Z. Extracellular superoxide dismutase, a molecular transducer of health benefits of exercise. Redox Biology May 2020;32:101508.

100 Woods JA. et. al. Exercise, inflammation and aging. Aging Dis. 2012 Feb;3(1):130–140.

101 Davis JM, Kohut ML, Colbert LH. Exercise, alveolar macrophage function, and susceptibility to respiratory infection. J Appl Physiol. 1985;83(5):1461-1466.

102 Benatti FB, Pedersen BK. Exercise as an anti-inflammatory therapy for rheumatic diseases-myokine regulation. Nat Rev Rheumatol. 2015;11(2):86-97.

103 Inciardi RM, Lupi L, Zaccone G, et al. Cardiac involvement in a patient with coronavirus disease 2019 (Covid-19) JAMA Cardiol. 2020;10.1001/jamacardio.2020.1096.

104 Martin SA, Pence BD, Woods JA. Exercise and respiratory tract viral infections. Exerc Sport Sci Rev. 2009;37(4):157-164.

105 Lowder T, Padgett DA, Woods JA. Moderate exercise protects mice from death due to influenza virus. Brain Behav Immun. 2005;19(5):377-380.

106 Rooney BV, Bigley AB, LaVoy EC, et al. Lymphocytes and monocytes egress peripheral blood within minutes after cessation of steady state exercise: a detailed temporal analysis of leukocyte extravasation. Physiol Behav. 2018; 194:260-267.

107 Powers SK, Bomkamp M, Ozdemir M, et al. Mechanisms of exercise-induced preconditioning in skeletal muscles. Redox Biol. 2020:101462.

108 Bowden KA, Davies, Pickles S, Sprung VS. et al. Reduced physical activity in young and older adults: metabolic and musculoskeletal implications.Ther Adv Endocrinol Metab. 2019;10.

109 Kruger K, Mooren FC, Pilat C. The immunomodulatory effects of physical activity. Curr Pharmaceut Des. 2016;22(24):3730-3748.

110 Li LQ, Huang T, Wang YQ, et al. Novel coronavirus patients' clinical characteristics, discharge rate, and fatality rate of meta-analysis. J Med Virol. 2019.

111 Schuler L, Cosgrove A. The New Rules for Lifting for Abs. Penguin Random House; 2012.

112 Cramer et al. Yoga in women with abdominal obesity— a randomized controlled trial. Dtsch Arztebl Int. Sep 2016;113(39): 645–652.

113 Cahn BR, et al. Yoga, Meditation and mind-body health: increased BDNF, cortisol awakening response, and Altered inflammatory marker expression after a 3-month yoga and meditation retreat. Front Hum Neurosci. 2017; 11:315.

114 (Mover et al. Stress-induced Cortisol Response and Fat Distribution in Women. Obes Res. May 1994;2(3):255-62. doi: 10.1002/j.1550-8528.1994.tb00055.x.

115 Abbott R, Lavretsky H. Tai chi and qigong for the treatment and prevention of mental disorders. Psychiatr Clin North Am. Mar 2013;36(1):109–119.

116 Pedersen BK. The diseasome of physical inactivity and the role of myokines in muscle fat cross talk. J Physiol 2009;587:5559–68.

117 Elffers et al. Body fat distribution, in particular visceral fat, is associated with cardio-metabolic risk factors in obese women. PLoS One. 2017;12(9):e0185403.

118 Jacobs et al. Waist circumference and all-cause mortality in a large US cohort. Arch Intern Med. 2010;170(15):1293-1301. doi:10.1001/archinternmed.2010.201.

119 Osterberg EC, Bernie AM, and Ramasamy R. Risks of testosterone replacement therapy in men. Indian J Urol. Jan-Mar 2014;30(1): 2–7.

120 Kraemer et al. The effects of short-term resistance training on endocrine function in men and women. Eur J Appl Physiol Occup Physiol. Jun 1998;78(1):69-76. doi: 10.1007/s004210050389.

121 Sato et al. Responses of Sex Steroid Hormones to Different Intensities of Exercise in Endurance Athletes. Exp Physiol. Jan 2016;101(1):168-75. doi: 10.1113/EP085361. Epub 2015 Dec 9

122 Pilz et al. Effect of vitamin D supplementation on testosterone levels in men. Horm Metab Res. Mar 2011;43(3):223-5.

123 Forrest K, Stuhldreher WL. Prevalence and correlates of vitamin D deficiency in US adults. Nutr Res. Jan 2011;31(1):48-54. doi: 10.1016/j.nutres.2010.12.001.

124 Wong et al. Effects of folic acid and zinc sulfate on male factor subfertility: a double-blind, randomized, placebo-controlled trial. Fertil Steril. Mar 2002;77(3):491-8. doi: 10.1016/s0015-0282(01)03229-0.

125 Chandrasekhar K, Kapoor J, Anishetty S. A prospective, randomized double-blind, placebo-controlled study of safety and efficacy of a high-concentration full-spectrum extract of ashwagandha root in reducing stress and anxiety in adults. Indian J Psychol Med. Jul 2012;34(3):255-62.

126 Ahmad et al. Withania Somnifera Improves Semen Quality by Regulating Reproductive Hormone Levels and Oxidative Stress in Seminal Plasma of Infertile Males. Fertil Steril Aug 2010;94(3):989-96.

127 Rains et al. A Randomized, Controlled, Crossover Trial to Assess the Acute Appetitive and Metabolic Effects of Sausage and Egg-Based Convenience Breakfast Meals in Overweight Premenopausal Women. Nutr J. Feb 10, 2015;14:17. doi: 10.1186/s12937-015-0002-7.

128 Vieira Senger AE, Schwanke CHA, Gomes I, Valle Gottlieb MG. Effect of green tea (Camellia sinensis) consumption on the components of metabolic syndrome in elderly. Journal of Nutrition, Health & Aging, Online First™. July 20, 2012.

129 Holt-Lunstad J, Smith TB, Layton JB. Social relationships and mortality Risk: a meta-analytic review.

130 Buettner D. Blue zones. National Geographic. 2010.

131 Dimsdale JE. Psychological stress and cardiovascular disease. J Am Coll Cardiol. 2008 Apr 1;51(13):1237–1246.

132 Yancy et al. Comparison of group medical visits combined with intensive weight management vs group medical visits alone for glycemia in patients with type 2 diabetes: a noninferiority randomized clinical trial. JAMA Intern Med. 2020;180(1):70-79. doi:10.1001/jamainternmed.2019.4802.

133 Musa-Veloso K, et al. Breath acetone is a reliable indicator of ketosis in adults consuming ketogenic meals. Am J Clin Nutr. 2002 Jul;76(1):65-70. doi: 10.1093/ajcn/76.1.65.

134 Wallace TM, et al. The hospital and home use of a 30-second hand-held blood ketone meter: guidelines for clinical practice. Diabet Med. Aug 2001;18(8):640-5. doi: 10.1046/j.1464-5491.2001.00550.x.

135 Gibson AA et al. Do ketogenic diets really suppress appetite? a systematic review and meta☐analysis. Obesity Reviews. Jan 2015;16(1):64-76.

136 Kondo et al. Vinegar intake reduces body weight, body fat mass, and serum triglyceride levels in bbese japanese subjects. Biosci. Biotechnol. Biochem. 2009;73(8):1837–1843.

137 Yancy et al. Comparison of group medical visits combined with intensive weight management vs group medical visits alone for glycemia in patients with type 2 diabetes: a noninferiority randomized clinical trial. JAMA Intern Med. 2020;180(1):70-79. doi:10.1001/jamainternmed.2019.4802.

138 Sacks et al. Dietary fats and cardiovascular disease: a presidential ddvisory from the American Heart Association. Circulation. Jul 2017;136(3, 18):e1-e23.

139 Gomez-Arbelaez et al. Acid–base safety during the course of a very low-calorie-ketogenic diet. Endocrine. 2017; 58(1):81–90.

140 Lustman P Clouse R. Depression in diabetic patients: The relationship between mood and glycemic control. J Diabetes and its Complications. Mar–Apr2005;19(2):113-122.

141 Meira et al. Ketogenic Diet and epilepsy: what we know so far. Front Neurosci. 2019;13:5.

142 Bough K. Energy metabolism as part of the anticonvulsant mechanism of the ketogenic diet. Epilepsia. 2008;49(Suppl. 8): 91–93.

143 Bostock et al. The current status of the ketogenic diet in psychiatry. Frontiers in Psychiatry. 2017;8:43.

144 Vogelzhangs N et al. Anxiety disorders and inflammation in a large adult cohort. Transl Psychiatry. Apr 2013; 3(4): e249.

145 Maes M. Depression is an inflammatory disease, but cell-mediated immune activation is the key component of depression. Progress in Neuro-Psychopharmacology and Biological Psychiatry. Apr 2011;35(3, 29):664-675.

146 Schagen SK, Zampeli VA, Makrantonaki E, Zouboulis CC. Discovering the link between nutrition and skin aging. Dermatoendocrinol. Jul 1,2012;4(3):298–307.

147 Rawlings AV. Ethnic skin types: are there differences in skin structure and function? Int J Cosmet Sci. 2006;28:79–93.

148 Makrantonaki E, Bekou V, Zouboulis CC, Genetics and skin aging. Dermatoendocrinol. 2012 Jul 1;4(3):280–284.

149 Palma L, Marques LT, Bujan J, and Rodrigues LM. Dietary water affects human skin hydration and biomechanics. Clin Cosmet Investig Dermatol. 2015;8:413–421.

150 Danby FW. Nutrition and aging skin: sugar and glycation. Clin Dermatol. Jul-Aug 2010;28(4):409-11. doi: 10.1016/j.clindermatol.2010.03.018.

151 Smith RN, Mann NJ, Braue A, et al. The effect of a high-protein, low glycemic-load diet versus a conventional, high glycemic-load diet on biochemical parameters associated with acne vulgaris: a randomized, investigator-masked, controlled trial. J Am Acad Dermatol. 2007;57(2):247–256.

152 Emma Weiss and Rajani Katta. Diet and rosacea: the role of dietary change in the management of rosacea. Dermatol Pract Concept. Oct 2017;7(4):31–37.

153 Constantin. Significance and impact of dietary factors on systemic lupus erythematosus pathogenesis. Exp Ther Med. Feb 2019;17(2):1085–1090.

154 Weisman MH. Inflammatory Back Pain. Rheum Dis Clin North Am. 2012 Aug; 38(3):501–512.

155 Khanna S, Jaiswal KS, Gupta B. Managing rheumatoid Arthritis with dietary interventions. Front Nutr. 2017; 4: 52.

156 Maroon JC, et al. Natural anti-inflammataory agents for pain relilef. Surg Meurol Int.2010; 1:80. Published online Dec 13, 2010.doi: 10.4103/2152-7806.73804.

157 Davis A. The dangers of NSAIDs: look both ways. Br J Gen Pract. 2016 Apr;66(645):172–173.

158 Wu at al. Soy food intake and circulating levels of inflammatory markers in chinese women. J Acad Nutr Diet. Ju2012 1;112(7): 996–1004.e4.doi:10.1016/j.jand.2012.04.001.

159 Santarelli RL, Pierre F, Corpet DE. Processed meat and colorectal cancer: a review of epidemiologic and experimental evidence. Nutr Cancer. 2008;60(2):131-44.

160 Topiwala A. Moderate alcohol consumption as risk factor for adverse brain outcomes and cognitive decline: longitudinal cohort study. BMJ 2017;357 doi: https://doi.org/10.1136/bmj.j2353.

161 de Visser, R. O., Robinson, E., & Bond, R. Voluntary temporary abstinence from alcohol during "Dry January" and subsequent alcohol use. Health Psychology. 2016;35(3):281–289. https://doi.org/10.1037/hea0000297.

162 Ebrahim IO1, Shapiro CM, Williams AJ, Fenwick PB. Alcohol and sleep I: effects on normal sleep. Alcohol Clin Exp Res. Apr 2013;37(4):539-49. doi: 10.1111/acer.12006. Epub 2013 Jan 24.

163 Romeo J, Wärnberg J, Nova E, Díaz LE, Gómez-Martinez S, Marcos A. Moderate alcohol consumption and the immune system: a review.Br J Nutr. Oct 2007;98 Suppl 1:S111-115.

164 Afshar et al. Acute immunomodulatory effects of binge alcohol ingestion. Alcohol. 2015 February;49(1):57-64.

165 Simet SM, Sisson JH. Alcohol's wffects on lung health and immunity. Alcohol Res. 2015;37(2): 199–208.

166 Husain K, Ansari RA, Ferder L. Alcohol-induced hypertension: mechanism and prevention. World J Cardiol. May 26, 2014;6(5):245–252.

167 Watenabe H. Beneficial biological effects of miso with reference to radiation injury, cancer and hypertension. J Toxicol Pathol. Jun 2013;26(2):91–103.

168 Clemente et al. The impact of the gut microbiota on human health: an integrative view. Cell. Mar 16, 2012; 148(6):1258–1270.

169 Buettner Dan. The Blue zones solution: eating and living like the world's healthiest people. National Geographic. 2017.

170 Willcox Bradley J, Willcox Craig D, and Suzuki Makoto. The Okinawa Diet Plan: Get Leaner, Live Longer, and Never Feel Hungry. Three Rivers Press; 2004

171 Richardson S, Hirsch JS, Narasimhan M. Crawford JM, McGinn T, Davidson KW. Presenting characteristics, comorbidities, and outcomes among 5700 patients hospitalized With Covid-19 in the NewYork City area. JAMA. Apr 22, 2020. doi: 10.1001/jama.2020.6775.

172 Centers for Disease Control Weekly Update. Provisional Death Counts for Coronavirus Disease 2019 (COVID-19) from August 26, 2020. Retrieved from, https://www.cdc.gov/nchs/nvss/vsrr/covid_weekly/index.htm

173 Ioannidis J. The infection fatality rate of Covid-19 inferred from seroprevalence data. medRxiv.

174 Franceschi C., Bonafè M., Valensin S., et al. Inflamm-aging. An evolutionary perspective on immunosenescence. Annals of the New York Academy of Sciences. 2000;908:244–254.

175 Xia S. et al. An update on inflamm-aging: mechanisms, prevention, and treatment. J Immunol Res. 2016; 2016: 8426874.

176 Morgan TE. et al. Anti-inflammatory mechanisms of dietary restriction in slowing aging processes. Interdiscip Top Gerontol. 2007;35:83-97.

177 Bonafe M, et al. Inflamm-aging: Why older men are the most susceptible to SARS-CoV-2 complicated outcomes. Cytokine & Growth Factor Reviews June 2020;53:33-37.

178 Szarc vel Szic K, et al. From inflammaging to healthy aging by dietary lifestyle choices: is epigenetics the key to personalized nutrition? Clinical Epigenetics. 2015;7:article number 33.

179 Rao, G, Rowland K. Zinc for the common cold—not if, but when. J Fam Pract. Nov 2011;60(11):669–671

180 Mayer K. HRE's number of the day: coronavirus stress. Human Resource Executive. Apr 14,2020.

181 Phillips JM, Clark C, Herman-Ferdinandez L, Moore-Medlin T, Rong X, Gill JR, Clifford JL, Abreo F, Nathan CO. Curcumin inhibits skin squamous cell carcinoma tumor growth in vivo. Otolaryngol Head Neck Surg. Jul 2011;145(1):58-63. doi: 10.1177/0194599811400711.

182 Heng MCY (2017) Topical Curcumin: A Review of Mechanisms and uses in Dermatology. Int J Dermatol Clin Res 3(1):010-017.

183 Stewart MG, Witsell DL, Smith TL, Weaver EM, Yueh B, Hannley MT. Development and validation of the Nasal Obstruction Symptom Evaluation (NOSE) Scale. Otolaryngol Head Neck Surg. February 2004;130:157-163.

184 Lanza DC, & Kennedy DW. Adult rhinosinusitis defined. Otolaryngol Head Neck Surg.1997;117(3):S1-S7. doi: 10.1016/S0194-59989770001-9.

185 Hamilos DL. Chronic rhinosinusitis: Epidemiology and medical management. J Allergy Clin Immunology. 2011;128(4): 693–707. doi: 10.1016/j.jaci.2011.08.004.

186 Fokkens WJ et al EPOS 2012European position paper on rhinosinusitis and nasal polyps 2012. Rhinology. 2012 Suppl.23:1-299. doi: 10.4193/Rhino50E2.

187 Sahebkar A, Henrotin Y. Analgesic efficacy and safety of curcuminoids in clinical practice: a systematic review and meta-analysis of randomized controlled trials. Pain Med. Jun 2016;17(6):1192-202.

188 Agrawal KA et al. Efficacy of turmeric (curcumin) in pain and postoperative fatigue after laparoscopic cholecystectomy: a double-blind, randomized placebo-controlled study. Surg Endosc. Dec 2011;25(12):3805-10.